Pathophysiology of the Human His-Purkinje System

Editor

MASOOD AKHTAR

CARDIAC ELECTROPHYSIOLOGY CLINICS

www.cardiacEP.theclinics.com

Consulting Editors
RANJAN K. THAKUR
ANDREA NATALE

December 2016 • Volume 8 • Number 4

ELSEVIER

1600 John F. Kennedy Boulevard • Suite 1800 • Philadelphia, Pennsylvania, 19103-2899

http://www.theclinics.com

CARDIAC ELECTROPHYSIOLOGY CLINICS Volume 8, Number 4
December 2016 ISSN 1877-9182, ISBN-13: 978-0-323-47735-2

Editor: Stacy Eastman
Developmental Editor: Susan Showalter

Cardiac Electrophysiology Clinics (ISSN 1877-9182) is published quarterly by Elsevier Inc., 360 Park Avenue South, New York, NY 10010-1710. Months of issue are March, June, September, and December. Subscription prices are $205.00 per year for US individuals, $318.00 per year for US institutions, $225.00 per year for Canadian individuals, $359.00 per year for Canadian institutions, $285.00 per year for international individuals, $384.00 per year for international institutions and $100.00 per year for US, Canadian and international students/residents. To receive student/resident rate, orders must be accompanied by name of affiliated institution, date of term, and the signature of program/residency coordinator on institution letterhead. Orders will be billed at individual rate until proof of status is received. Foreign air speed delivery is included in all Clinics subscription prices. All prices are subject to change without notice. **POSTMASTER:** Send address changes to Cardiac Electrophysiology Clinics, Elsevier Health Sciences Division, Subscription Customer Service, 3251 Riverport Lane, Maryland Heights, MO 63043. **Customer Service: 1-800-654-2452 (US and Canada). From outside of the US and Canada, call 314-477-8871. Fax: 314-447-8029. E-mail: JournalsCustomerService-usa@elsevier.com (for print support); JournalsOnlineSupport-usa@elsevier.com (for online support).**

Reprints. For copies of 100 or more of articles in this publication, please contact the Commercial Reprints Department, Elsevier Inc., 360 Park Avenue South, New York, NY 10010-1710. Tel.: 212-633-3874; Fax: 212-633-3820; E-mail: reprints@elsevier.com.

Cardiac Electrophysiology Clinics is covered in *MEDLINE/PubMed (Index Medicus)*.

Contributors

CONSULTING EDITORS

RANJAN K. THAKUR, MD, MPH, MBA, FHRS
Professor of Medicine and Director, Arrhythmia
Service, Thoracic and Cardiovascular Institute,
Sparrow Health System, Michigan State
University, Lansing, Michigan

ANDREA NATALE, MD, FACC, FHRS, FESC
Texas Cardiac Arrhythmia Institute at
St. David's Medical Center, Austin,
Texas

EDITOR

**MASOOD AKHTAR, MD, FACC, FACP,
MACP, FAHA, FHRS**
Aurora Cardiovascular Services, Director of
Electrophysiology Research, Aurora
Sinai/Aurora St. Luke's Medical Centers,
Adjunct Clinical Professor of Medicine,
University of Wisconsin School of Medicine
and Public Health, Milwaukee, Wisconsin

AUTHORS

**MASOOD AKHTAR, MD, FACC, FACP,
MACP, FAHA, FHRS**
Aurora Cardiovascular Services, Director of
Electrophysiology Research, Aurora
Sinai/Aurora St. Luke's Medical Centers,
Adjunct Clinical Professor of Medicine,
University of Wisconsin School of Medicine
and Public Health, Milwaukee, Wisconsin

SAMUEL J. ASIRVATHAM, MD, FHRS
Professor; Cardiac Electrophysiologist, Mayo
Clinic, Rochester, Minnesota

ILKNUR CAN, MD
Professor, Department of Cardiology, Meram
School of Medicine, Necmettin Erbakan
University, Konya, Turkey

ANWER A. DHALA, MD, FACC, FHRS
Electrophysiologist, Aurora Cardiovascular
Services, Aurora Sinai/Aurora St. Luke's
Medical Centers; Clinical Professor of
Pediatrics, Pediatric Electrophyisiology,
Children's Hospital of Wisconsin, Medical
College of Wisconsin, Milwaukee, Wisconsin

SARFRAZ A. DURRANI, MD
MedStar Heart and Vascular Institute,
Fairfax, Virginia

WARREN M. JACKMAN, MD
George Lynn Cross Research Professor, Heart
Rhythm Institute, University of Oklahoma
College of Medicine, Oklahoma City,
Oklahoma

MOHAMED KANJ, MD
Department of Cardiovascular Medicine,
Cleveland, Ohio

MELVIN SCHEINMAN, MD
University of California San Francisco Medical
Center, San Francisco, California

ANOOP K. SINGH, MD, BCh
Program Director, Pediatric Cardiac
Electrophysiology Services; Assistant
Professor, Children's Hospital of Wisconsin,
Medical College of Wisconsin, Milwaukee,
Wisconsin

RAPHAEL SUNG, MD
Peninsula Primary Care - Cardiology, Medical Director of Community Hospital's Section of Cardiac Electrophysiology, Monterey, California

KHALDOUN TARAKJI, MD, MPH
Department of Cardiovascular Medicine, Cleveland, Ohio

PATRICK TCHOU, MD
Department of Cardiovascular Medicine, Cleveland, Ohio

VENKATAKRISHNA N. THOLAKANAHALLI, MD, FHRS
Associate Professor of Medicine; Staff Cardiac Electrophysiologist, Minneapolis VA Health Care System, University of Minnesota, Minneapolis, Minnesota

Contents

Part I

The His-Purkinje system (HPS) plays a significant role in human pathophysiology, but knowledge is scattered. This article highlights some of the relevant concepts, phenomena, and mechanisms; clarifies, expands, confirms, or modifies commonly encountered clinical events; and adds new information, which is often available but obscure. Also included are the essentials of HPS anatomy and physiology. It is important to abandon inaccurate concepts that are still taught and occasionally appear in text books.

Part II

This review covers many of the arrhythmias and conduction abnormalities related to His-Purkinje System. These include junctional premature complexes, junctional and fascicular tachycardias, bundle branch reentry (BBR), and the role of apparent conduction in various forms of supraventricular tachycardias (SVT) with or without involvement of accessory pathways (AP).

Part III (Cases)

The patient exhibits multiple features suggestive of Timothy syndrome, which is a multisystem autosomal-dominant condition with findings that include prolonged QT interval, hand and foot abnormalities, dysmorphic facial features, and mental retardation. A 2:1 infranodal atrioventricular block may occasionally be seen in the setting of severely prolonged QT interval. Functional nature of atrioventricular block is demonstrated by resumption of 1:1 conduction with changes in heart rate.

A single beat arising as extra systole within the His-Purkinje system or from ventricle or even atrium based on conduction timing can invoke delayed conduction or block within intra-Hisian or infra-Hisian sites. This may be either manifested in the form of premature atrial or ventricular complexes or concealed as with His extra systoles. It appears commonly there is disease within the His-Purkinje system.

Bidirectional Ventricular Tachycardia Due to a Mixture of Focal Fascicular Firing and Reentry

Sarfraz A. Durrani, Raphael Sung, and Melvin Scheinman

Bidirectional ventricular tachycardia (BDVT) is a well-known phenomenon since it was first described in 1922. Various mechanisms have been proposed for BDVT, including digitalis toxicity, hypokalemia, Anderson-Tawil syndrome, acute myocarditis, and catecholaminergic polymorphic ventricular tachycardia. It is characterized by rapid, wide complex electrocardiogram pattern with alternating QRS morphology and axis. The alternation of the QRS is usually right bundle branch block with 180° swings in the frontal plane axis or, less commonly, alternation of right bundle branch and left bundle branch forms. Most of the proposed mechanisms involve triggered activity or enhanced automaticity. We describe a unique BDVT, with characteristics of both re-entry and triggered activity, which terminated with a focal Rf lesion.

Recording the *Accessory His Bundle Potential* from a Right Atriofascicular Accessory Pathway

Warren M. Jackman

The author discusses the case of a 42-year-old man with a long history of episodes of rapid palpitations. Recordings from the proximal end of a right atriofascicular accessory pathway at the lateral tricuspid annulus are discussed. There was successful catheter ablation of the right atriofascicular accessory pathway, without recurrence of tachycardia.

Wenckebach Phenomenon in the His-Purkinje System

Masood Akhtar

The author discusses Wenckebach phenomenon (WP) in the His-Purkinje system (HPS). Subtle PR changes may be interpreted as no change, often seen in the HPS-WP. Changes in the QRS axis help to localize the site of delay and block along fascicles of the left bundle branch. Marked PR changes may occur during HPS-WP. All the QRS complexes that are conducted depict right bundle branch and left anterior superior fascicular block, so the visible changes in the HV interval suggest WP mostly occurring in the left posterior inferior fascicle.

Wenckebach Phenomenon in Left Bundle Branch Block

Masood Akhtar

A 60-year-old patient had recurrent wide QRS complex tachycardia with a left bundle branch and normal axis pattern. The underlying mechanism was atrioventricular nodal reentry tachycardia. Besides the palpitation, there were no other symptoms. The cardiovascular examination was normal.

Retrograde Concealed Conduction in the His-Purkinje System

Masood Akhtar

An 83-year-old man was seen due to recurrent syncopal episodes. Only the His bundle recording was able to be obtained, which showed the His-Purkinje System as the site of a conduction delay. A permanent dual-chamber pacemaker was implanted with no further syncopal episodes.

Changes in the Reentrant Pathway in Verapamil-Sensitive Fascicular Reentrant Ventricular Tachycardia During Ablation

Patrick Tchou, Khaldoun Tarakji, and Mohamed Kanj

The sequence of changes in the QRS morphology and the accompanying cycle lengths of the tachycardia confirm that the reentrant circuit involves the left ventricular myocardium as well as the His Purkinje system as part of the reentrant circuit. The reentrant propagation likely goes from local left ventricular myocardium into a slowly conducting, verapamil-sensitive tissue, which then connects into the inferior fascicle. This case demonstrates that fascicular reentrant tachycardias can generate different QRS morphologies depending on the path of breakout into the myocardium.

CARDIAC ELECTROPHYSIOLOGY CLINICS

ISSUE OF RELATED INTEREST

Critical Care Nursing Clinics, September 2016 (Vol. 28, No. 3)
Cardiac Arrhythmias
Mary G. Carey, *Editor*
Available at: http://www.ccnursing.theclinics.com/

THE CLINICS ARE AVAILABLE ONLINE!
Access your subscription at:
www.theclinics.com

Foreword

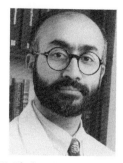
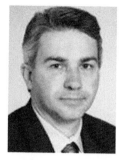

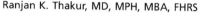

Ranjan K. Thakur, MD, MPH, MBA, FHRS   Andrea Natale, MD, FACC, FHRS, FESC

Consulting Editors

Before I came here I was confused about this subject. Having listened to you, I am still confused, but on a higher level.
         —Enrico Fermi

The His-Purkinje system was discovered in the 19th century, and it was recognized that it was responsible for swift conduction of the electrical impulse from the atrium to the ventricle, allowing for synchronous depolarization of both ventricles. Over the years, our understanding of physiology and pathology of the His-Purkinje system has evolved, but we are still refining our understanding about arrhythmias and arrhythmia mechanisms. As a case in point, in the early 1990s, we used to talk about "idiopathic left ventricular tachycardia" or ILVT, originating from the mid-septal left ventricle as a unique arrhythmia. Soon thereafter, the broader concept of fascicular ventricular tachycardias was appreciated and ILVT was recognized as one form of fascicular ventricular tachycardia.

The His-Purkinje system has been shown to play a central role in many electrophysiologic disorders encountered in practice. First, it was recognized that a diseased His-Purkinje system may lead to atrioventricular conduction disorders resulting in bradycardias. The His-Purkinje system is also necessary for perpetuation of both typical and atypical forms of atrioventricular re-entrant tachycardias as well as bundle branch re-entry and fascicular ventricular tachycardia. More recently, automaticity in the His-Purkinje system has been found to be responsible for the initiation and perpetuation of focal ventricular tachycardia and,

more ominously, ventricular fibrillation in otherwise normal hearts.

In this issue of the *Cardiac Electrophysiology Clinics*, Dr Masood Akhtar is guiding us through the physiology and pathology of the His-Purkinje system relevant for clinicians, illustrated with clinical cases covering all aspects of this essential structure. Dr Akhtar is impeccably qualified for this contribution, having described many physiologic concepts regarding the His-Purkinje system as well as clinical arrhythmias originating in the conduction system.

This issue of the *Cardiac Electrophysiology Clinics* should be required reading for all electrophysiology fellows in training and clinicians in practice. We hope that the readers will enjoy reading it and find it useful in enhancing their understanding of clinical arrhythmias originating in the His-Purkinje system.

Ranjan K. Thakur, MD, MPH, MBA, FHRS
Sparrow Thoracic and Cardiovascular Institute
Michigan State University
1200 East Michigan Avenue, Suite 580
Lansing, MI 48912, USA

Andrea Natale, MD, FACC, FHRS, FESC
Texas Cardiac Arrhythmia Institute
at St. David's Medical Center
3000 North I-35, Suite 720
Austin, TX 78705, USA

E-mail addresses:
thakur@msu.edu (R.K. Thakur)
dr.natale@gmail.com (A. Natale)

Card Electrophysiol Clin 8 (2016) ix
http://dx.doi.org/10.1016/j.ccep.2016.09.002
1877-9182/16/© 2016 Published by Elsevier Inc.

Preface

Pathophysiology of the Human His-Purkinje System

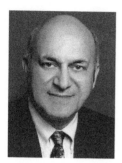

Masood Akhtar, MD, FACC, FACP, MACP, FAHA, FHRS
Editor

For some uncertain reasons, medical literature is replete with writing about normal and abnormal sinoatrial node, atria, atrioventricular node, and ventricular myocardium. This cannot be stated with certainty regarding the human His-Purkinje system (HPS).

In this issue of *Cardiac Electrophysiology Clinics*, an attempt is made to explore the physiology and abnormality that often prompts a visit to the physician. The understanding of normal human HPS and its response to various external maneuvers helps to distinguish when it is abnormal. Part 1 of the issue is devoted to physiology, whereas Part 2 deals with cardiac conduction abnormalities and tachycardias, which either originate from HPS or are part of presentation, often making for diagnostic difficulties. The interpretation of some complex arrhythmias could be intellectually challenging and may require additional data to make an accurate diagnosis.

This issue is designed to help serious students of clinical cardiac electrophysiology better understand the HPS, which will lead to satisfaction, more knowledgeable interpretation, and better patient care. While the material contained here is available in some form or another, the intent was to make it available in one compact format, and I hope that is partially achieved.

Masood Akhtar, MD, FACC, FACP, FAHA, FHRS
Aurora Cardiovascular Services
Aurora Sinai/Aurora St. Luke's Medical Centers
University of Wisconsin School of Medicine
and Public Health
2801 West Kinnickinnic River Parkway
Suite 777
Milwaukee, WI 53215, USA

E-mail address:
publishing@aurora.org

http://dx.doi.org/10.1016/j.ccep.2016.09.001
1877-9182/16/© 2016 Published by Elsevier Inc

ardiacEP.theclinics.com

Part I

Part I

Human His-Purkinje System
Normal Electrophysiologic Behavior

Masood Akhtar, MD, FACC, FACP, MACP, FAHA, FHRS

KEYWORDS

- Trifascicular left bundle branch • His-Purkinje system • Bundle branches • Phenomena of gap
- Linking, gating, and impulse integration • Accessory pathways

KEY POINTS

- The left bundle branch has 3 divisions, and the septal division is functional both in the anterograde and retrograde directions.
- In individuals with normal baseline His-Purkinje system (HPS), all of the phenomena (ie, bundle branch block, HV prolongation, and complete block in the HPS are normal events with premature stimuli.
- Many of the physiologic properties of the HPS (ie, conduction, refractory periods) are similar in anterograde and retrograde directions.
- A thorough study of the HPS requires additional recordings from the bundle branch or fascicles.
- Whether some of the details here are necessary for good patient care may be debatable; however, knowledge of these concepts is important to understand and meet the minimal teaching standards of electrophysiology for a good foundation.

INTRODUCTION

During atrioventricular (AV) conduction, several anatomic structures are traversed by the supraventricular impulse to reach the ventricular myocardium (VM), initiating ventricular contraction, the most important event in the process. These components are sinoatrial (SA) tissue, atria, atrioventricular node (AVN), His bundle, bundle branches, Purkinje network (the His-Purkinje system [HPS]), Purkinje VM junction, and the VM. In the clinical literature, HPS physiology and its role in clinical arrhythmias is infrequently discussed, scattered, and mostly studied during the propagation of electrical impulses in the anterograde direction.[1–7] AV nodal conduction and refractory periods (RPs) generally exceed that of the HPS, so the abnormal HPS lends itself for evaluation. The use of atrial pacing, manipulation of pacing cycles and occasionally spontaneous cycle length (CL) change caused by atrial and ventricular premature complexes, and long pauses allow the study of the HPS.[6–10] At times, it is necessary to use certain pharmacologic agents, such as low-dose atropine (0.5 mg), to facilitate AV nodal conduction in order to unmask the electrophysiologic properties of the HPS or resort to ventricular pacing to achieve that goal.[11]

With better understanding of arrhythmias arising from the ventricle, and other infranodal and extranodal structures such as accessory pathways (APs), the role of the HPS has taken on greater importance.[12–15] In the retrograde direction, as seen with ventricular tachycardia (VT), fully preexcited QRS complexes, and ventricular pacing, the ventricular impulse encounters the HPS directly.[16–18] The AVN therefore does not pose

Aurora Cardiovascular Services, Aurora Sinai/Aurora St. Luke's Medical Centers, University of Wisconsin School of Medicine and Public Health, 2801 W. Kinnickinnic River Parkway, Suite 777, Milwaukee, WI, USA
E-mail address: publishing@aurora.org

Card Electrophysiol Clin 8 (2016) 641–682
http://dx.doi.org/10.1016/j.ccep.2016.07.003
1877-9182/16/© 2016 Elsevier Inc. All rights reserved.

an impediment, as it does in the anterograde direction, and this has further expanded the understanding of the HPS. Even though intracardiac electrophysiology has improved comprehension of the HPS, a lot of this literature remains obscure and is seldom incorporated in the interpretation of simple, as opposed to complex, arrhythmias. This article presents the current understanding of the human HPS (its practical anatomy, pathophysiology, and role in clinical arrhythmias).

PRACTICAL ANATOMY

Wilhelm His, Jr. at Leipzig, Germany, described the bundle that carries his name in 1893[19] and Jan E. Purkinje had already published his work in 1839.[20] For convenience, the entire infranodal specialized conduction tissue (ie, the His bundle [HB], bundle branches [BB], fascicles, and the Purkinje network) is collectively referred to here as the HPS. Normally, the HB per se does not give out branches until it divides into the thin right bundle branch (RBB) and much larger left bundle branch (LBB). Although the RBB has a somewhat uniform course along the right side of the interventricular septum, the LBB has a more variable and complex anatomy. Kulburtus and Demoulin[21] described the variation of human LBB anatomy in clear terms in 49 human hearts (**Fig. 1**). The most common pattern, which they called type 1, shows a clear septal (centroseptal) division, (ie, a third division), which in some cases was the largest compared with the anterior (superior) and posterior (inferior) fascicles. In 17 of 49 cases the septal division originated directly from the main left bundle (LB). In another 9 cases, the septal division branched from the left posterior fascicle, whereas in 7 cases it came off the anterior division. Because of the

trifascicular nature of LBB, the term hemiblock is avoided in this article and fascicular or divisional block is used instead, as suggested by Hecht HH and colleagues, Dhala A and colleagues, and Sung RK and colleagues.[22–24]

Some clinical electrophysiologic and electrocardiogram (ECG) evidence helps to support the concept of the trifascicular LBBB (LBBB).[23,24] This topic is discussed later for fascicular tachycardias and preablation and postablation (RB) scenarios. However, without the existence and active role played by the septal fascicle, some tachycardias and conduction patterns could not be satisfactorily explained.[23,24]

At this juncture, it is important to point out that disorder of the LBB may or may not produce a cause and effect relationship (with physiology) in a given clinical situation. Even when the two (ie, anatomy and pathophysiology) correlate qualitatively, the extent of clinical manifestation may not. Isolated HPS disorder, although more common in the elderly, does not spare the younger population, and HPS-related tachycardias may occur in patients with normal VM function and valves, as discussed later. Embryologic developments of HPS and related abnormalities in pediatric populations are outside the scope of this article.

Pathologic states can affect the HPS when there is extensive disease such as idiopathic or ischemic cardiomyopathy; Chagas disease; or, at times, small lesions such as fibrosis or calcium deposits. Fibrosis and calcium deposits are more common in association with valvular disease, the HPS is quite compact (ie, the HB and proximal BB). In certain instances, the HPS may be the only affected tissue responsible for patients' symptoms.

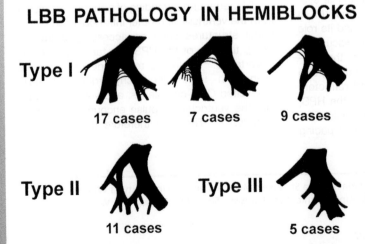

LBB PATHOLOGY IN HEMIBLOCKS

Type I   17 cases   7 cases   9 cases

Type II   11 cases   **Type III**   5 cases

Fig. 1. Anatomy of left bundle branch showing the main left bundle (LB) and its division from 49 human hearts. In 31 of the 49 patients the LB had a distinct third division originating from the main LB, its posterior inferior fascicle, or anterior superior fascicle. The variety of LB distribution in the 3 types of patterns can be appreciated. Several patients with the 3 types of patterns are shown. See text for more details. (*From* Kulbertus HD, Demoulin JCL. Pathological basis of concept of left hemiblock. In: Wellens HJJ, Lie KI, Janse MJ, editors. The conduction system of the heart: structure, function and clinical implications. New York: Springer; 1978. p. 289; with permission.)

After division of the HB, 3 or 4 fascicles emerge in various anatomic formats (**Fig. 2**), spread out as the Purkinje network, which penetrates the VM from the endocardial to the epicardial direction. Therefore, at a given time, a small unit of VM is depolarized while the current flows rapidly along the subendocardial Purkinje network. Breakthrough of the impulse from 4 different points (ie, the 3 fascicles of the LBB and RBB) occurs almost at the same time. Combined with simultaneous activation of the 2 ventricles is what produces the so-called normal QRS, with a duration of 60 to 100 milliseconds. Note that normal QRS is not synonymous with narrow QRS. Although normal QRS must be narrow, it also has a certain orientation in 3 dimensions, as observed on a 12-lead ECG. In contrast, a narrow QRS complex may not be normal. For example, there may be a Q wave infarct and minimal or no associated prolongation of QRS duration.

His-Purkinje System Recording with Electrode Catheter

By providing a marker between the atria and ventricles, recordings of HB potential have markedly increased the comprehension of the AV junction.[1] It is usually done by placing an electrode catheter across the tricuspid valve (generally 1 mm to 1 cm interelectrode spacing). Shorter interelectrode distance (1–2 mm) provides a better definition of HB potential with less contamination from the local atrial and ventricular electrograms. HB deflection

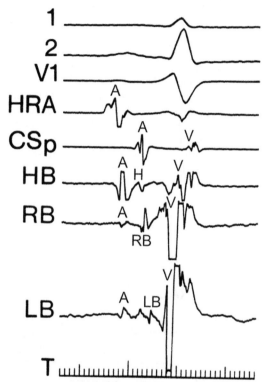

Fig. 3. Catheter recording of proximal HPS. The tracings from top to bottom are surface ECG I, II, and V1. High right atrium (HRA), proximal coronary sinus (CSp), His bundle (HB), right bundle (RB) and LB branch recordings, respectively, and T (timelines) at 10 to 100 milliseconds. Simultaneous recording from the HB, RB, and LB are seldom available and require at least 2 electrode catheters (ie, on either side of interventricular septum). Typically, 3 surface ECGs are concurrently recorded. The intracardiac recordings are filtered differently and not used for P wave or QRS complex morphology, but are used in the timing and sequence of electrophysiologic events; hence the directionality of impulse propagation. The BB recordings are identified by a shorter interval; typically RB-V or LB-V less than or equal to 30 milliseconds with minimal or no atrial electrogram. When possible, RB should be recorded as distal as possible as long as it is recognizable. Although not labeled, the measurements are HV = 40 milliseconds, RB-V = 20 milliseconds, and LB-V = 20 milliseconds. The sequence of atrial activation is high to low, typical of sinus rhythm. Similar abbreviations are used in subsequent tracings unless indicated otherwise. All intracardiac intervals are measured in milliseconds.

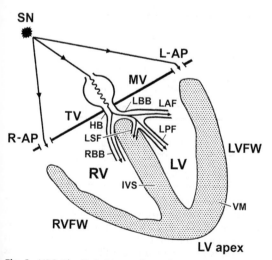

Fig. 2. HPS. The 3 divisions of LBB that exist in most individuals. This diagram shows LBB with 3 rather than 2 fascicles. IVS, interventricular septum; LAF, left anterior superior fascicle; L-AP, left free wall accessory pathway; LPF, left posterior inferior fascicle; LSF, left septal fascicle; LV, left ventricle apex; LVFW, left ventricular free wall; MV, mitral valve; R-AP, right free wall accessory pathway; RFW, right ventricular free wall; RV, right ventricle; SN, sinoatrial node; TV, tricuspid valve.

can also be recorded from the left side of the interventricular septum just below the aortic valve. RB potential is recordable by simply advancing the HB recording catheter. From a single, quadripolar, or multipolar electrode catheter both HB and RB potential can be recorded. If both HB and distal RB potential recordings are desirable, it will require 1 multipolar electrode catheter or 2 catheters. Some catheter manipulation is often required to obtain a satisfactory recording. Similarly, electrical potential from the anterior and posterior divisions of the LBB or the main LB can be recorded by the transaortic approach. These recordings are helpful in understanding complex arrhythmias arising from the HPS, for both the nature of the circuit and directionality of impulse propagation, particularly when the LBB and/or its divisions are involved (**Fig. 3**).

Routine recordings from the left side are seldom performed, and it may not be necessary to record both HB and BB potentials in most narrow complex tachycardias. During a wide QRS tachycardia, the absence of BB recording and sole reliance on HB timing and QRS morphology may not be sufficient and can be misleading. This possibility applies both in physiologic and pathologic situations, particularly in the presence of anterograde functioning AP (ie, ventricular preexcitation). Examples of this are given later.

Just as important is electrical stimulation of various cardiac chambers to replicate conduction abnormalities and induction of previous documented or suspected cardiac arrhythmias.[25] The critical importance of electrical stimulation cannot be understood until it is realized that almost all abnormal rhythms being sought are not present at the time of the study. The growth of clinical cardiac electrophysiology can be credited to the discovery of intracardiac recordings as well as programmed electrical stimulation.[1,25]

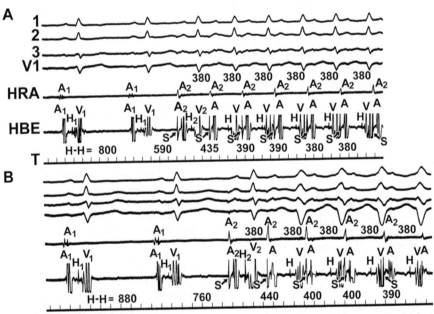

Fig. 4. HPS response to constant CL atrial pacing. During sinus rhythm A_1A_1 (*A*, *B*) constant CL atrial pacing is initiated at 380 milliseconds (A_2A_2). Both the atrial and H-H CL are labeled. (*A*) The A_1A_2 coupling (sinus to first paced atrial complex; S_1 denotes stimulus artifact) is 590 milliseconds preceded by 800 milliseconds and conducts normally. With the second A_2, the A_2H_2 is prolonged, which in turn prolongs the H-H CL to 435 milliseconds, whereas atrial pacing is still 380 milliseconds. CL of 435 milliseconds represents 73% of the previous CL of 590 milliseconds and so does not encroach on the refractoriness of HPS, and conducts normally, as do all of the remaining atrial paced complexes. During this random onset of pacing, the A_1A_2 (*B*) is 760 milliseconds, which is followed by 440 milliseconds, which is 57% (ie, 760–440 milliseconds of A_1A_1). Relative shortening of H-H in this case approaches the refractoriness of LBB and results in LBBB pattern. Continuation of the LBBB pattern is caused by retrograde invasion of LBB reaching the LV via the RBB and then transseptally to LBB, which creates an area refractory to the next anterograde impulse (ie, retrograde concealed conduction, penetration, or linking phenomenon in LBB). The continuation of the LBB pattern is caused by repetition of the same. The key factor that differs in the two panels is the change from A_1A_2 to the next A_2A_2 intervals. (*From* Damato AN, Varghese PJ, Caracta AR, et al. Functional 2:1 AV block within the His-Purkinje system: simulation of type II second degree AV block. Circulation 1973;47:540; with permission.)

Further description of HPS behavior is outlined later. The terms normal, physiologic, and/or functional are defined by 4 main criteria in this article: (1) the individual does not have any symptoms related to the HPS or tachycardia with HPS participation; (2) the baseline QRS morphology, HPS conduction times, and RPs are normal and respond normally to pacing; (3) the HPS response to cardioactive drugs is within expected normal limits; and (4) the observed electrophysiologic finding does not require any medical treatment.

The presence of an AP per se may be considered abnormal; however, normal versus abnormal AP behavior has never been clearly defined. Furthermore, the HPS physiology in patients with AP has not been described as different compared with individuals without AP.[26,27] Henceforth the mere coexistence of AP with a normal pathway

(NP) is described in physiologic terms. Vague terms such as weak AP and so forth are not used here.

NORMAL HIS-PURKINJE SYSTEM (PHYSIOLOGY)
Response of His-Purkinje System During Anterograde Impulse Propagation

During anterograde propagation, the HPS conduction time (the so-called HV interval) measures 35 to 55 milliseconds (see **Fig. 3**). With gradual acceleration of the heart rate, such as during exercise, and/or constant CL atrial pacing at a faster rate, in which the first paced beat has a long coupling interval (**Fig. 4A**)[a] the HV remains unchanged, as does the subsequent QRS width and morphology, because

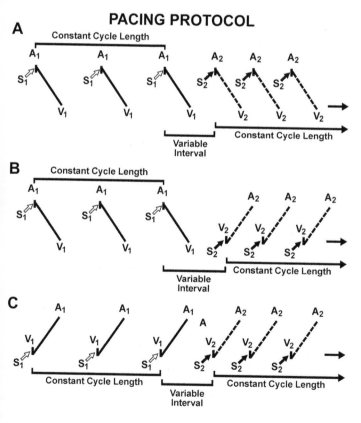

PACING PROTOCOL

Fig. 5. Sudden CL change and HPS (pacing design). The pacing protocol used to study HPS response to sudden CL change. To avoid CL variation during sinus and random-onset pacing (see **Fig. 4**), a specific protocol was designed. The initial or basic CL and pacing site (first train) designated S_1S_1 (*white arrows*), A_1A_1, or V_1V_1 is followed by a variable coupling interval to the second train S_2S_2 (*black arrows*), A_2A_2, V_2V_2, which were also kept at constant but shorter CL. The interval between the first and second train is labeled as coupling interval S_1S_2, A_1A_2, (A) A_1V_2 (B) and V_1V_2 (C) were varied but all deliberately chosen and different coupling intervals were examined. In many cases only 1 CL of the second train was introduced (ie, 1 A_2A_2, V_2V_2 at a time). The response of HPS to the first A_2A_2 or V_2V_2 was fully assessed before the second CL of the second train was introduced. This sequence was maintained until a stable state was reached. (*Adapted from* Akhtar M, Lehmann MH, Denker ST, et al. Electrophysiologic mechanisms of orthodromic tachycardia initiation during ventricular pacing in the Wolff-Parkinson-White syndrome. J Am Coll Cardiol 1987;9:90; with permission.)

---

[a]It is customary to denote sinus or constant atrial CL pacing as S_1 or A_1 with S representing stimulus artifact. The label S_2A_2 is used to describe the atrial premature complexes. Similar abbreviations are used for ventricular pacing (eg, S_1V_1 S_2V_2). When a deviation in protocol takes place for a specific study, it is outlined in the methods or explained in the legend, as is done in this article.

the HPS appropriately shortens its refractoriness (sometimes referred to as accommodation).

With further but gradual shortening of the CL, such as in sinus tachycardia during exercise, no change in the HV or QRS is expected up to maximum heart rate.

The same happens during incremental pacing and 1:1 AV conduction down to a CL of 300 milliseconds. A change in the coupling interval (see **Fig. 4**B), and/or at a CL less than 300 milliseconds, or a sudden rate acceleration may produce different results (**Figs. 5** and **6**).[27] A systematic study to assess the anterograde HPS response to CL shorter than 300 milliseconds has not been carefully examined.

To properly examine HPS behavior during a gradual increase in heart rate, the pacing protocol has to simulate the gradual CL shortening seen

with exercise, without the concomitant sympathetic stimulation or parasympathetic withdrawal, or both, because catecholamines per se could influence HPS properties unless autonomic blockade is done during the evaluation. Personal observations using a similar pacing protocol (without autonomic blockade) have suggested that HPS conduction delay and/or block with a gradual decrease in CL is not a normal response until proved otherwise. As a general rule, atrial pacing impulses start showing delay and/or block in the AVN before HPS refractoriness is reached. Once an atrial impulse blocks in the AVN the resulting H-H CL is prolonged and the next atrial impulse responds to a long H-H followed by a shorter H-H interval. Thus, aberrant conduction, prolonged HV with or without bundle branch block (BBB), and/or infra-Hisian block may ensue (see

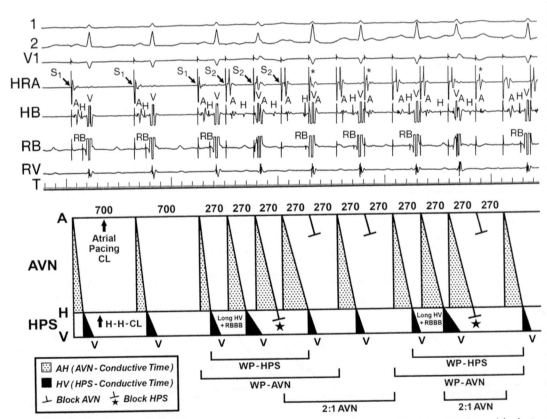

Fig. 6. Sudden atrial CL change and HPS. The tracing shows the protocol shown in **Fig. 5**A in a patient with electrograms with sudden atrial CL change from 700 to 270 milliseconds, also shown in a detailed ladder diagram. The coupling interval (ie, S_1S_2) measures the same as S_2S_2 train. The first S_2 functions as an atrial premature complex with AH delay (AVN) on HB trace (*stippled triangle*) HV delay (*black triangle*) and RBBB pattern (surface ECG lead V1). The third S_2 blocks in the HPS (ie, H but no QRS) and is shown at the bottom, with block and a star (Wenckebach phenomenon [WP] HPS). Fourth, sixth, and tenth paced S_2 impulses block in the AVN and are shown by the asterisk or HRA (on HB A_2 is not followed by H). There is simultaneous second-degree block in the AVN and HPS (WP) ongoing at the same time and depicted in brackets at the bottom. Note that both HPS and Wenckebach cycle are preceded by long H-H cycles. The first is a spontaneously longer H_1H_1 and the second follows a long H-H caused by block of A_2 in the AVN (*second asterisk*). The rest of the tracing is a repeat of this pattern. (*Adapted from* Akhtar M, Mahmud R, Tchou PJ, et al. Normal electrophysiologic responses of the human heart. Cardiol Clin 1986;4:367; with permission.)

Fig. 6). This physiologic response of the HPS to sudden CL changes is expected and therefore not abnormal.

At some point during atrial pacing intra-atrial, AV nodal, and/or AV reentrant tachycardia may be induced. In the presence of a functioning AP in the anterograde direction (overt preexcitation), the HV interval (as measured from the onset of HB deflection to the onset of QRS on surface and/or intracardiac recording, whichever is earlier) is either shorter than normal (**Fig. 7**), nonexistent, or may have a negative value. Depending on the effective RP (ERP) of AVN-HPS (ie, the NP versus AP; see **Fig. 7**), incremental pacing (or atrial extra-stimulus; ie, A_2) results in progressive prolongation in AV nodal conduction time with little or no change in PR via the AP. This process produces a greater degree of preexcitation because of a larger contribution to ventricular depolarization via the AP (see **Fig. 7**).[2,5] The block of the atrial impulse in the AP often coincides with the onset of orthodromic tachycardia (anterograde conduction along the NP and retrograde via AP; **Fig. 8**),

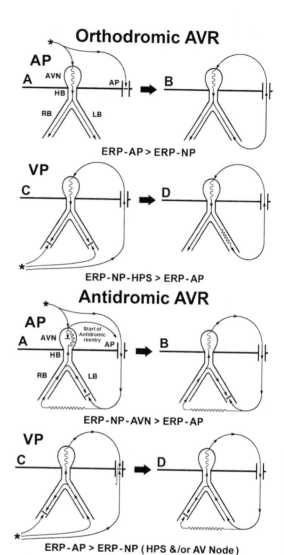

Fig. 8. Role of HPS in the onset of orthodromic and antidromic atrioventricular reentry (AVR). The usual mechanisms of orthodromic and antidromic AVR induction are shown. The mechanism of tachycardia onset with atrial pacing (*A*) and ventricular pacing (*C*) are self-explanatory, as is the continuation (*B, D*). Note that the so-called NP consists of AVN and HPS. The HPS conduction delay and/or block has a significant but different role in the 2 directions (ie, antero-grade and retrograde) on initiation or the lack thereof and the CL of tachycardia in all supraventricular tachycardia (SVT) using AV-AP because VM is an essential part of the reentry circuit. Depending on the RPs and recovery properties (AP vs AVN-HPS) both orthodromic and antidromic SVT can be preferentially initiated either from atria or ventricles. During antidromic reentry, retrograde ipsilateral BBB is deliberately created to highlight the role of the HPS and hence the CL of the circuit; this happens in the anterograde direction as well, but that is more widely appreciated. *, pacing site.

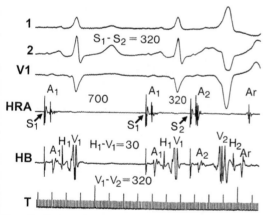

Fig. 7. HPS and ventricular preexcitation. During paced atrial CL of 700 milliseconds (A_1A_1) a single premature atrial complex (A_2) is introduced. The baseline H_1V_1 is shorter than normal and measures 30 milliseconds (normal, 35–55 milliseconds). The A_2 delays and/or blocks in the AVN. The resulting QRS is fully preexcited (H_2 comes after V_2). Noteworthy points are (1) there is no delay along the AP (ie, $A_1A_2 = V_1V_2$) and both V_1V_2 activates first through the AP (short HV and ventricular preexcitation); and (2) the activation route via the AP is maintained during V_2. The H_2 is followed by retrograde atrial activation (Ar) with short HA interval. The phenomenon seen in this tracing may represent anterograde activation of V_2 via the AP followed by H_2 through the NP or a result of V_1V_2 via the AP (like ventricular pacing). It can also be interpreted as A_2H_2 through the AVN and then atrial reciprocal beat (ie, caused by AV nodal reentry).

particularly if NP conduction is prolonged concomitantly allowing a longer time for AP recovery from prior impulse penetration. Because the onset of orthodromic tachycardia depends on AV delay rather than AV nodal delay (ie, HPS delay in addition), the HV prolongation or ipsilateral BBB (corresponding with the ventricle where the AP inserts; **Fig. 9**) also provides additional delay for AP recovery.[28] This situation can be better appreciated with a single atrial extrastimulus (see **Fig. 9**).[28] In contrast, if the atrial impulse blocks in the AVN but conducts anterograde via the AP, several types of preexcited tachycardia can be initiated that also involve the HPS. **Fig. 8** only shows 1 form, called antidromic AV reentry, in which the reentry circuit is the reverse of the orthodromic counterpart.

Unlike the HPS response to a gradual increase in heart rate (an abrupt change in CL; ie, to a premature atrial complex), the HPS frequently manifests conduction delays and/or block, depending on the coupling interval and duration of previous CL (**Fig. 10**).[16,29,30] As a general guide, physiologic HPS conduction delay can be observed when the premature H-H interval is less than or equal to 65% to 70% of the preceding H-H CL (at CL >400 milliseconds) because of impulse encroachment on the relative RP (RRP) of HPS. In the study of aberrant conduction, (ie, BBB, fascicular block, or both), it is important to realize that QRS morphology, axis, and so forth is the end result of the impulse propagation through the HPS (**Fig. 11**).[29] The key factor is the H-H CL preceding the aberrant QRS complex, and it is

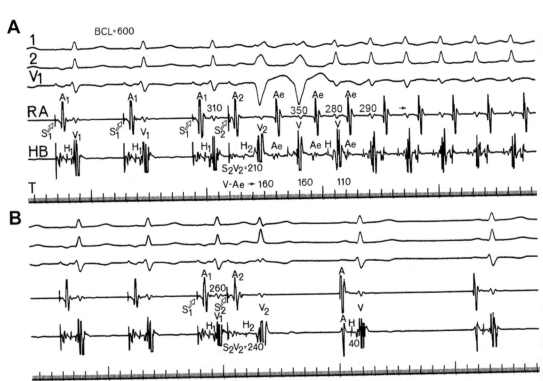

Fig. 9. HPS and induction of AVR. At a basic CL of 600 milliseconds and A_1A_2 of 310 milliseconds the A_2 conducts with S_2V_2 of 210 milliseconds (ie, S_2H_2 plus H_2V_2) and LBBB pattern. Sustained orthodromic AV reentry is initiated. (*B*) Despite a shorter A_1A_2, and longer S_2V_2 of 240 milliseconds, no tachycardia is induced. Although there is no evidence of AP during atrial pacing or sinus rhythm, left free wall AP conducting (concealed AP) retrograde can be diagnosed. Owing to LBBB, there is transseptal conduction delay added to the S_2V_2 interval to reach the AP. This delay is clearly evident from the V-A duration of 160 milliseconds with aberrant complex compared with normal QRS complex (110 milliseconds). These 50 milliseconds (difference in VA interval) when added to S_2V_2 are sufficient for AP recovery of excitability to conduct retrograde to the atria and start the SVT (*A*). This process can be deduced from the tracing in spite of the lack of coronary sinus (left atrial) recording. BCL, basic CL. (*From* Akhtar M, Lehmann MH, Denker S, et al. Role of His-Purkinje system in the initiation of orthodromic tachycardia in Wolff-Parkinson White syndrome. In: Benditt DG, Benson DW, editors. Cardiac preexcitation syndromes. New York: Martinus Nijhoff Publishing (Springer); 1986. p. 144; with permission.)

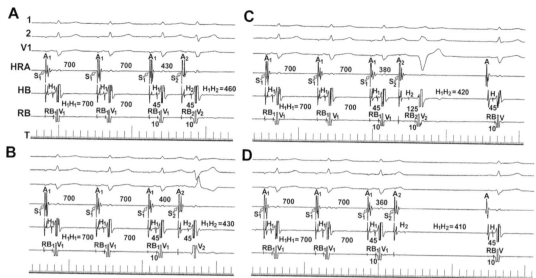

Fig. 10. HPS response to single atrial extrastimulus. The basic CL is 700 milliseconds (*A–D*). The atrial coupling (A_1A_2) is progressively shortened from 430 to 360 milliseconds. The corresponding H_1H_2 is labeled. (*A*) Minor superior axis shift, whereas at shorter H_1H_2 there is a combination of RBBB and left anterior superior fascicular block pattern (bifascicular block) in B. Conduction via the posterior inferior fascicles remains normal, so the H_2V_2 remains normal at 45 milliseconds. Note the disappearance of RB_2 deflection in B caused by conduction delay and/or block between H_2 and RB_2 in B. Further shortening of the H_1H_2 LBBB pattern and normal axis is observed. Also, the H_2V_2 is prolonged (125 milliseconds) and RB_2 reappears because now ventricular activation is through the RBB and the conduction delay is proximal to RB and distal to HB, $RB_2 V_2$ interval is the same (10 milliseconds) as sinus beats (last complexes in C and D) as well as during the basic drive. Further abbreviation of H_1H_2 results in infra-Hisian block (ie, no QRS in D) and the site of block continues to be between the H_2 and RB_2 recording sites. Note that despite shorter H_1H_2 in C versus in B, the V_1V_2 (R_1R_2) in C (465 vs 430 milliseconds) is longer because of marked H_2V_2 prolongation indicating concurrent RBBB and/or intra-HB delay.

not recorded on the surface ECG, so accurate timing of HB activation must be considered for definitive diagnosis. This point is emphasized in the schema (see **Fig. 11**) of aberrant conduction as seen on surface ECG (panel A) and then highlighted with HB location (panel B), and this relationship between the H and QRS is shown in a patient during the scanning of a basic CL with progressively shorter atrial coupling intervals (**Fig. 12**).

Once the RRP of the HPS is encountered, it manifests as a BBB, fascicular block, HV prolongation, or various combinations. All of the phenomena discussed earlier are considered physiologic and are observed in the setting of normal baseline intraventricular conductions (see **Fig. 10**). They are more readily shown during atrial bigeminy because it creates a scenario of longest followed by the shortest achievable H-H CL (**Fig. 13**).[30] The H-H CL following the premature complex is the so-called return or escape H-H CL, which is the longest achievable in a normal individual and exceeds sinus H-H CL. This CL in turn is followed by the next premature atrial complex, thus allowing the setting of the longest H-H

followed by the shortest H-H interval (discussed later).

The physiologic HPS events in spontaneous clinical settings are seldom captured because of the limited time of recording. Furthermore, the spontaneous onset of a clinical arrhythmic event is rarely observed even during electrophysiologic evaluation. However, in the laboratory setting, AV conduction, including HPS behavior, can be evaluated during pacing, manipulation of pacing cycles, and sometimes with a small amount of atropine (0.05 mg).[11] Atropine exerts no direct effect on the HPS but shortens refractoriness of AVN. The study of the HPS during sinus rhythm creates CL variations, hence pacing at CL just shorter than sinus CL allows constancy, consistency, and reproducibility, which is a more acceptable scientific approach.[26,27] Hence much of what is presented here occurs during pacing rather than sinus rhythm.

Although constant CL pacing is often referred to as incremental pacing, the randomness of coupling of the first paced complex to the prior spontaneous atrial complex functions as a

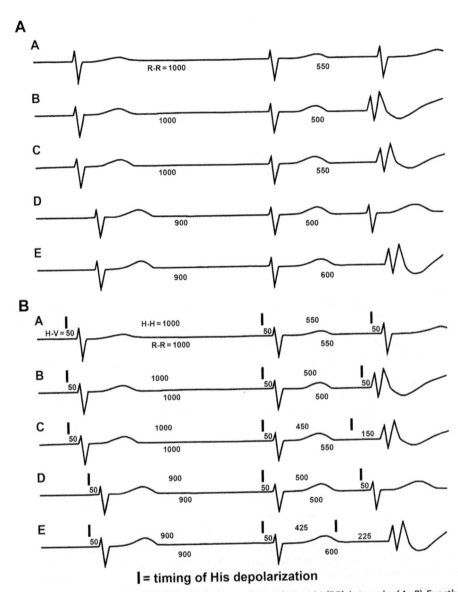

I = timing of His depolarization

Fig. 11. The cause and effect relationship between H-H and resultant VV (RR) intervals. (*A, B*) Exactly the same long and short CL, shown in milliseconds. The premature complexes are narrow or wide. The difference between the two panels is that A shows only surface ECG (RR intervals) and B shows projected timing of HB activation, thus RR, H-H, and HV intervals are shown. Without understanding of this relationship, tracings C and E in both panels can be misinterpreted as being of ventricular origin, but both are aberrant QRS complexes. Note also that **Fig. 10B** and C and also **Fig. 12** show the H to QRS relationship in the patient, which draws attention to the limitation of surface ECG interpretation.

premature beat that in turn determines the HPS response (**Figs. 14** and **15**).[31,32] This beat changes the HPS behavior depending on the H_1H_1 CL, duration of H_1H_2 coupling, and the CL of the subsequent train of pacing. Unless properly timed to previous sinus CL (which is not done routinely), the so-called incremental pacing acts as a series of premature impulses. To

prevent the obvious shortcoming of routine incremental pacing, the authors designed a pacing protocol to control the site of pacing duration of basic CL, coupling interval, and the CL and pacing site of the next train. This pacing design permitted a more systematic study of HPS physiology, which is presented in this article (see **Fig. 5**).[32]

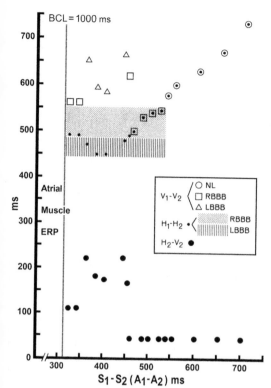

Fig. 12. Interplay between HPS and ventricular activation. At a BCL of 1000 milliseconds, A_1A_2 intervals are plotted against the various events shown in the box and measured in milliseconds. This scanning of BCL with progressively shorter A_1A_2 in a patient shows that until A_1A_2 of 560 milliseconds, the $H_1H_2 = V_1V_2$, because there is no H_2V_2 prolongation. However, the QRS begins to show an RBBB pattern at A_1A_2 of 550 milliseconds. The H_2V_2 prolongation with RBBB or LBBB is noted at all H_1H_2 of 450 milliseconds or shorter in an unpredictable fashion. At an H_1H_2 of 450 milliseconds, the V_1V_2 interval exceeds H_1H_2 by almost 200 milliseconds with LBBB pattern. During all of the symbols above the hatched area the V_1V_2 intervals exceed corresponding H_1H_2 intervals with either RBBB or LBBB pattern. NL, normal. (*From* Denker S, Gilbert CJ, Shenasa M, et al. An electrocardiographic-electrophysiologic correlation of aberrant ventricular conduction in man. J Electrocardiol 1983;16:274; with permission.)

Initial Site of Block in the His-Purkinje System and Downstream Impulse Migration

During anterograde propagation of atrial premature complexes in patients with baseline normal HPS, the site of conduction delay and/or block in the HPS is proximal, including in those patients with concealed AP as defined by electrophysiologic criteria, not ECG criteria (ie, no ventricular preexcitation regardless of the location of atrial impulse origin).[33] The site of block can be shown by a recording of the HB and proximal BB recordings at least on the right side (ie, H-RB interval prolongation; **Figs. 16–19**).[8] This observation is true with the first premature complex (A_2) because with the second (A_3) and subsequent premature complexes (S_4, and so forth) the site of block shifts distal to the RB recording site (see **Fig. 17**). This distal migration of the site of block is the most common mechanism for spontaneous resolution of BBB, even when it occurs during regular rates (see **Fig. 19**).

Linking Phenomenon and Resolution of His-Purkinje System Block

BBB occurs despite distal migration it can be sustained over 2 or more CLs for a variable period of time. The postulated mechanism for this phenomenon is often referred to as the linking phenomenon (**Figs. 20–23**).[34,35] With anterograde BBB the impulse travels to the ventricles via the contralateral BB and, after transseptal conduction, retrogradely penetrates into the anterogradely blocked BB. Hence the ipsilateral BB is refractory to the next oncoming supraventricular impulse.[34]

Alternate terms have been used for this mechanism of repeated functional BBB despite a constant CL. These terms include repetitive retrograde concealed conduction or penetration. Linking is more inclusive and unifies diverse phenomena currently carrying other terminologies. For example, sustained BBB at constant CL and entrainment of all tachycardias (ie, AVN reentrant tachycardia, bundle branch reentry [BBR], and scar-related VT) all have the linking phenomenon as an essential requirement for their occurrence. The initial role of linking in maintaining BBB or entrainment is important to even comprehend the electrophysiology of these events. Some examples are shown in **Figs. 21–23**. It is also critical to understand that the 2 impulses outlined in the linking process are from 2 different generations: the previous with the current or current with the future. The present impulse is designated as n and prior impulse as n−1, whereas the next is n + 1, as shown in **Fig. 20**.

Reentrant circuits have been visualized in which the head of the reentrant impulse is chasing the tail of the previous current with the excitable gap in between. The existence of this excitable gap makes the entrainment possible because, without excitable gap during reentry, entry into the circuit, entrainment, and even termination with pacing is not possible. Note that the concept of linking by collision in a physiologic human model has also been shown, and it is a prerequisite before the entrainment is even possible in any reentrant circuit.[33,34]

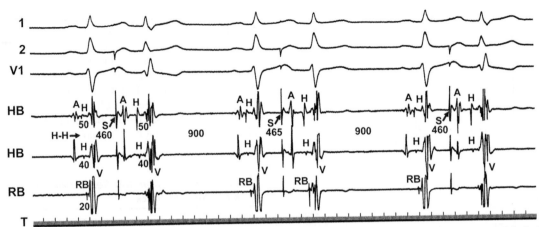

Fig. 13. Atrial bigeminy and HPS. Sinus and atrial premature complexes are alternating. The H-H CLs are labeled. The first atrial premature complex results in longer A-H, no change in HV interval, and an RBBB pattern. Note that the RB-V interval, which measures 20 milliseconds during sinus, is now not measurable because RB potential cannot be recognized as a result of delay between the H and RB potentials. The RB potential is either merged into the corresponding V electrogram because of conduction delay or there is a block between the H and RB recording sites. The next H-H CLs (both proximal and distal) shorten because the AH (ie, AV nodal conduction time) is prolonged after the premature complex. The RB-RB is even shorter because (1) if H_2 conducts to RB then RB is obscured by the QRS, or (2) if a block occurred between H & RB then retrograde penetration will further delay RB activation and this will result in even greater RB-RB CL shortening. Consequently, the second premature complex conducts normally; the RB deflection returns; the RB-RB is longer again, similar to the first premature complex; and the next atrial premature complex again shows a repeat the same phenomenon and the return of RBBB.

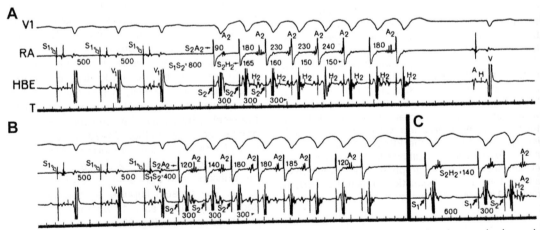

Fig. 14. HPS response to sudden change in CL. This response corresponds with the protocol example shown in Fig. 5B (A_1–V_2 change). The basic atrial CL (for first train, only the last 3 S_1 depicted) is 500 milliseconds in both panels. In A the first S_2 follows a long CL of 800 milliseconds and conducts with no delay in either the AVN (ie, HA) or HPS (VH), the A_2 on HBE is obscured in the corresponding V electrogram, and the S_2A_2 is 90 milliseconds on the RA electrogram. Subsequent S_2A_2 V_2V_2 are all 300 milliseconds. The second S_2 behaves like an early premature ventricular complex; retrograde blocks in the RBB and reaches H_2 via LBB, and starts linking in the RBB. V_2H_2 stabilizes at 150 milliseconds and is preceded by a subtle HA (AVN) WP and then 2:1 block (no A_2 after sixth and eighth paced S_2 in both [A] and [B]). By shortening the coupling of S_1S_2 to 400 milliseconds (B) there is immediate 1:1 HPS accommodation with no delay. However, there is HA-WP and 2:1 HA block, as in A, because as far as the AVN is concerned the second train CL (ie, 300 milliseconds) is the same as (A). (C) Reference cycle showing the emergence of H_2 from V_2 with ventricular pacing during the basic CL of 600 milliseconds. (*From* Lehmann MH, Denker S, Mahmud R, et al. Functional His-Purkinje System behavior during sudden ventricular rate acceleration in man. Circulation 1983;68:771; with permission.)

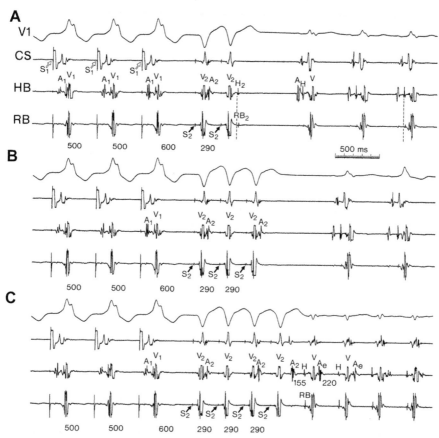

Fig. 15. Response of HPS and AP to sudden CL change. The pacing design is the same as in **Fig. 14** and **Fig. 5**B (ie, the change from atrial to ventricular pacing train). The difference is that this patient has a left free wall AP, and only 1 cycle of S_2S_2 train is introduced at a time. The CL of the first train (A_1A_1) is 500 milliseconds, the coupling A_1V_2 at 600 milliseconds (A–C) of second train V_2V_2 is 290 milliseconds in all panels, but only 1 CL is introduced at a time. Pacing is from the coronary sinus (CS) (first train) and RV (second train). Fully preexcited QRS complexes are noted during CS pacing compared with sinus rhythm (at the end of panels A and B) because pacing is close to the atrial insertion of AP. The AV interval is short and H_1 is buried in the local V_1 electrogram. Because of the long S_1S_2 (V_1V_2), the first ventricular paced complex in all panels shows no conduction delay (short $V_2 A_2$) because of longer S_1V_2. The second V_2 acts as an early premature ventricular complex and conducts along the NP to activate H_2 via the NP but blocks in the AVN and in AP (no A_2). The second ventricular premature complex is added in B, but in this case S_2 blocks in the HPS and AP (no H_2 or A_2). The second S_2 activates through AP and NP like the first S_2. (C) Another S_2 is added, which blocks in the HPS and conducts via AP (ie, A is activated before the H). The atrial impulse that occurred via the AP now has no impediment in the NP and conducts to the ventricle to initiate orthodromic AV reentry. The first AH is shorter than the next, confirming that the S_2 that started the tachycardia never reaches the AVN (ie, it is blocked in the HPS).

Eventually, the linking phenomenon can abolish spontaneously or intentionally by several mechanisms. (1) Spontaneous or induced ventricular premature complex ipsilateral or contralateral to the BBB (or site of linking) by retrograde penetration and shortening of the refractoriness of involved BB (ie, peeling back of the RP) (**Fig. 24**). The events in **Fig. 24** are too complex to explain normalization of QRS by pacing in the contralateral ventricle. Linking by collision has to occur in RBB and the same premature impulse probably blocks in the LBB distal to the linking site by interference, and terminates. (2) Blocked atrial premature complexes, which prolong the return cycle, causing longer H-H CL, which is outside the RP of the BB, thus abolishing the BBB.[27] (3) Similarly, rate variations during atrial fibrillation often produce sufficiently long R-R (H-H) intervals, which can exceed the RP of the BB, resulting in normalization of QRS (**Fig. 25**).[35,36] (4) Although primarily studied in a retrograde direction with a systematic pacing protocol, the HPS displays a damped oscillatory

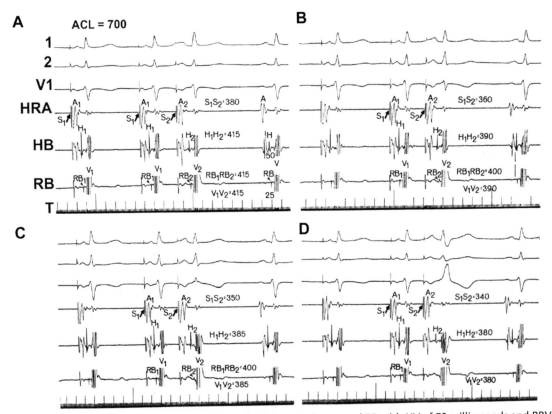

Fig. 16. Proximal site of block HPS. During sinus rhythm both the HB and RB with HV of 50 milliseconds and RBV of 25 milliseconds (with HRB interval of 25 milliseconds) are shown and can be clearly appreciated. An A_1A_2 decrease from A and D at basic atrial paced CL (ACL) of 700 milliseconds are labeled. Progressive prolongation of the H_2-RB_2 interval is noted from B to C along with a change in QRS configuration on the surface ECG, particularly in lead V_1. Further delays between H_2 and RB_2 (*D*) result in RB_2 deflection either merging into local V_2 electrogram or there is a block of H_2 impulse. The same proximal delay can also be observed in **Figs. 10** and **13**. (*From* Akhtar M, Gilbert CJ, Al-Nouri M, et al. Site of conduction delay during functional block in the His-Purkinje system in man. Circulation 1980;61:1241; with permission.)

pattern, which may be another reason for spontaneous disappearance of aberrant conduction (**Fig. 26**).[37] This is discussed again later in the context of ventricular pacing. (5) However, the most common mechanism for spontaneous resolution of functional BBB is distal migration and can be shown without activation of the ventricle (see **Figs. 17–19** and **21**). Most spontaneous episodes of nonsustained aberrancy do not require premature complexes; a frequent occurrence in the laboratory setting, where spontaneous resolution of aberrant conduction is common.

Site of Distal His-Purkinje System Block and Gating Phenomenon

The finding of proximal location of block in the HPS following first atrial premature complex and migration downstream (distal to the most distal RB recording) during the subsequent atrial pace complex is different compared with the gating phenomenon in the experimental animal models.[38] The gating in that setting shows progressive prolongation of the action potential duration (APD) from proximal to peripheral HPS. This prolongation implies that the distal Purkinje network has the longest RP and functions as a gate for supraventricular impulses to reach VM. A proper comparison may not be possible because (1) multiple recordings along the HPS have seldom been done in humans; and (2) in a physiologic setting, proximal block only applies to various fascicles with the first premature atrial complex. Subsequent atrial paced complex at a similar CL block distally, caused by impulse migration most probably caused by shortening of local RP at the site of block; (3) in a small percentage of cases (around 10%) the initial HPS block is distal to the RB

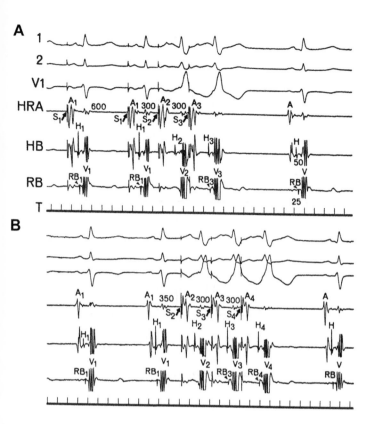

Fig. 17. Proximal to distal migration in HPS. Same patient as **Fig. 16**. Two extrastimuli (A_2A_3) at basic atrial paced CL of 600 in A, and 3 (A_2A_3 and A4) during sinus rhythm (*B*) are shown. Note that the site of block along the RBB has moved from proximal (between H_2 and RB_2) to distal (RB_3, RB_4) locations beyond the RB recording site. The H_3 RB_3, RB_3-V_3, RB_4-V_4 measures the same as sinus complexes. Also, QRS morphology during all complexes shows complete RBB pattern and corresponding HV intervals are all identical. (*Reproduced from* Akhtar M, Gilbert CJ, Al-Nouri M, et al. Site of conduction delay during functional block in the His-Purkinje system in man. Circulation 1980;61:1246.)

recording.[8] When a concomitant HV and H-RB delay is noted, it is assumed that a similar proximal conduction delay is also occurring along the LBB. However, direct recording from the proximal or distal LBB has not been done systematically in patients with normal HPS conduction at the baseline (as in **Fig. 3**). During retrograde propagation with ventricular pacing, antidromic reentry, the site of retrograde block is distal (ie, distal to the most distal RB recording; discussed later regarding retrograde conduction). It therefore seems that the initial site of functional block in human HPS is closest to the site of premature complexes. This statement is made with the caveat that incremental RP from proximal to distal HPS (or the reverse) in humans remains uncertain.

Ashman Phenomenon, Concealed Conduction His-Purkinje System, and Related Observations

Another aspect of HPS behavior is worth examining, popularized by and relating to the so-called Ashman phenomenon.[39] The observation was made that a long CL followed by a short CL (in the setting of atrial fibrillation) may conduct aberrantly if the short H-H CL encroaches on the RRP or ERP of a given BB. Such an aberrancy or HPS block is more complex, and identical long-short CL sequences may or may not be aberrant (**Fig. 27**).[40]

Although in the past ECG literature provided alternative explanations, systematic studies in the human HPS give a different answer.[41,42] It seems that the CL before the long CL has a profound effect on the HPS RP, and this was learned by designing a specific protocol. **Fig. 28** shows this graphically. Compared with constant CL as the reference point, the short-long-short sequence leads to HPS refractoriness that exceeds that of the long CL (**Fig. 29A–C**).[41] The opposite occurs (ie, HPS refractoriness decreases as the long CL is preceded by an even longer CL; see **Fig. 29D, E**).[41] This phenomenon cannot be explained from anticipated APD of the chosen CL alone, but instead the duration of the diastolic interval (**Fig. 30**)[42] (ie, the interval between the end of the previous to the onset of the next action potential, as shown in **Fig. 30**) provides a better explanation.[41] A short-long sequence leads to longer diastolic intervals to which the HPS response is prolongation of RRP-ERP, and the opposite happens with longer-long-short sequence compared with constant CL (see **Fig. 30**).

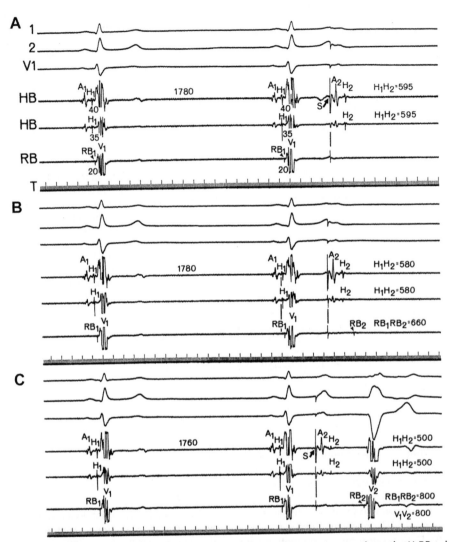

Fig. 18. HPS conduction delay, block, and gap phenomenon. All are shown to occur along the H-RB axis. The long CLs are all sinus and there is a proximal, distal HB and RB recording. There is a distal H to RB interval of 15 milliseconds at the baseline with an RB-V of 20 milliseconds. The A_1A_2 intervals progressively shorten from A to C. The corresponding H_1H_2 measure 595, 580, and 500 milliseconds, respectively. Note that in A the A_2 impulse blocks between the HB and RB (no RB deflection). The absence of QRS indicates concomitant block in the LBB system and/or in the HB. At shorter H_1H_2 (*B*) conduction resumes to RB_2 (ie, the impulse has slowed and migrated downstream to activate RB_2, but blocks beyond that). Marked conduction delay between H_2RB_2 of 300 milliseconds (*C*) results in effective propagation to the ventricle with LBBB pattern. This profound conduction delay between H and RB is a physiologic event in a patient with normal baseline conduction with an H-RB interval of 15 milliseconds during sinus but it is still less than what is happening along the H-LB axis (ie, QRS shows LBBB). (*Reproduced from* Akhtar M, Gilbert CJ, Al-Nouri M, et al. Site of conduction delay during functional block in the His-Purkinje system in man. Circulation 1980;61:1244; with permission; and Akhtar M, Sra JS. Physiological responses during electrophysiologic evaluation. In: Sra JS, Akhtar M, editors. Practical electrophysiology. Minneapolis (MN): Cardiotext; 2014. p. 60.)

Cycle Length Alternation and His-Purkinje System

As mentioned earlier, during atrial bigeminy, several HPS phenomena are observed that are not readily noticeable otherwise.[30] **Figs. 31** and **32** show paced atrial bigeminy in both, and the panels are not continuous.[30] The first 2 cycles in **Fig. 31** are constant at 750 milliseconds. Following that, there is a paced atrial bigeminy and

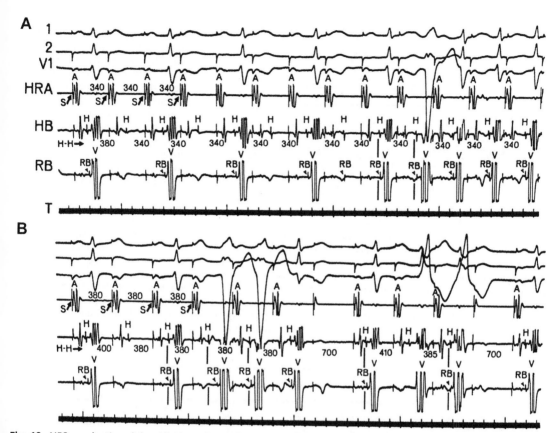

Fig. 19. HPS conduction delay, block, and impulse migration at constant CL pacing. A and B are not continuous. Constant paced atrial CL is 340 milliseconds and 380 milliseconds in A and B, respectively. Perpendiculars are drawn to indicate the H and RB relationship. During narrow QRS complexes, the H deflection clearly precedes the RB by 15 milliseconds. (*A*) A 2:1 block in the HPS between H and RB (no RB potential after H and no QRS) occurs after second, fourth, and sixth paced atrial complexes. Note that RB deflection reappears after H (eighth paced atrial complex) but blocks downstream, below the RB (no QRS). The 10th atrial paced complex conducts with LBBB and after that 1:1 conduction continues with narrow QRS complexes. (*B*) Even though there is HV and RBV prolongation preceding LBBB (compared with narrow QRS complexes), H-RB measures the same in B as narrow QRS complex. When 2:1 block is followed by 1:1 conduction the first complex also shows an LBBB pattern. Here the H-RB is prolonged before the QRS. The first aberrantly conducted QRS in A and B seems to behave differently. As is almost always the case with the first conducted complex (with the RBBB or LBBB), the HRB is prolonged. The complex in A seems to defy the rule, unlike the first complex with left or RBBB in B. The reason for this response is simple: the distal migration has already occurred during the 2:1 conduction with the eighth atrial paced complex, as pointed out earlier. Missed atrial capture and hence a long H-H (*B*) again initiates aberrant conduction that is, RBBB (*B*). As expected, there is an HRB delay with the first complex (no RB identified) but distal migration with the second identical QRS complex with RBBB. (*From* Akhtar M, Gilbert CJ, Al-Nouri M, et al. Site of conduction delay during functional block in the His-Purkinje system in man. Circulation 1980;61:1245; with permission.)

alternating 360 milliseconds and 750 milliseconds atrial CL. The H-H intervals are labeled and the relevant measurements are shown. At the HB level, the alternate cycles measure 660 and 450 milliseconds, except the first 2 CLs in panel A and the end of panel B, where the 2 CLs are constant at 750 milliseconds. Despite the paced and controlled, identical CLs of short and long sequence, the premature complexes show aberrant conduction (RBBB) alternating with normal

(NL) QRS (see **Fig. 32**). The first atrial premature in panel A (fourth QRS) is narrow, but the next is aberrant and this continues until the end in panel B, where the 2 constant CLs of 750 milliseconds are followed by a premature but NL QRS complex. What appears to be an unpredictable response has a logical explanation. When there is RBBB, some part of RBB gets activated later compared with the LBB. Additional retrograde penetration of the RBB via the LBB (linking phenomena) further

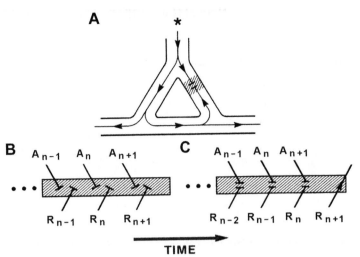

Fig. 20. Linking phenomenon. A universal event between the cardiac conducting tissue whenever there is more than 1 pathway. (*A*) Classic model of reentry. There is the initial site of block in one pathway, and propagation in the other, which reaches the site of block from the opposite direction. Depending on the state of recovery for excitability caused by prior activation, the two opposing impulses may continue to provide obstacles for each other once established. There are at least 2 mechanisms shown in B and C by which alternate impulses could link this way. (*A*) The so-called linking by interference. Black dots represent an ongoing process in which the hatched area explains the mechanism. The previous impulse (n-1) blocks but in its wake leaves an area around it that is partially depolarized. The next impulse from the opposite direction is unable to negotiate this area for continued propagation but leaves in its aftermath a residual area of refractoriness. This area in turn leads to block of the next impulse and the process of linking by interference continues. In contrast, linking by collision occurs in all reentrant circuits when a paced impulse can enter an excitable gap and conducts both orthodromically to reset and collide antidromically with the previous impulse on its way to where the paced impulse enters the circuit. Linking by interference is shown in B and linking by collision in C. Examples of linking by interference with intracardiac tracings are shown in **Figs. 21** and **22** and by collision in **Figs. 23** and **24**. See text for more details. *, origin of electrical impulse.

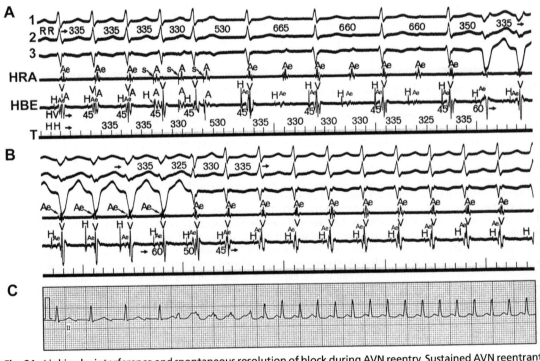

Fig. 21. Linking by interference and spontaneous resolution of block during AVN reentry. Sustained AVN reentrant tachycardia (AVN-RT) is shown in all panels. After 3 narrow QRS complexes with ongoing slow-fast AVN-RT, 3 atrial paced extrastimuli are introduced, which initiate a 2:1 block in the HPS (ie, H but no QRS), while the AV nodal AVN-RT continues. Note the short duration of the P wave caused by simultaneous activation of both atria. Near the end of panel A, the 1:1 AV relationship resumes. The first conducted QRS complex shows LBBB, which continues (*A* and *B* are continuous), but no significant change in the atrial CL of tachycardia. A transition from 2:1 to 1:1 AV conduction almost always results in aberrancy caused by uneven recovery of BB. The only logical explanation for continuation of LBBB despite the same CL as narrow QRS is retrograde concealed conduction into the LB via transseptal conduction from RBB, referred to from here on as linking (by interference). The site of linking migrates downstream and results in narrow QRS tachycardia. Note an incomplete LBBB complex sandwiched between the LBBB and narrow QRS complex (*C*). An ECG rhythm strip from another patient shows how a 2:1 block HPS, 1:1 conduction with LBBB, and narrow QRS complex (event seen in *A* and *B*) appear on the surface ECG rhythm strip.

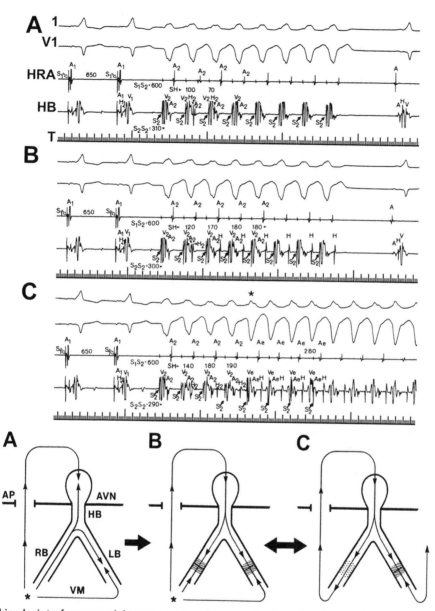

Fig. 22. Linking by interference and downstream impulse migration in patients with AP. Anterograde AV-AP conduction (ventricular preexcitation HV = 0) can be appreciated during sinus rhythm and atrial pacing at 650 milliseconds (A_1A_1). The A_1A_2 coupling is 600 milliseconds in all panels and the pacing design is (A_1-V_2) as shown in **Fig. 5**B. Only the S_2S_2 train CL is changed from 310 to 300 milliseconds and then 290 milliseconds in A, B, and C, respectively. The first S_2 conducts via both NP and AP but the retrograde H_2 is obscured by the V_2 electrogram. The second S_2 behaves like a premature complex and H_2 emerges but is difficult to identify because A_2 via the AP occurs at the same time, followed by quick accommodation (*top panel*) when both AP and NP conduct rapidly. (*B*) At S_2S_2 of 300 milliseconds there is retrograde HPS. WP (ie, rapid VH >slow VH > HPS block that occurs with the third S_2. Note that A_2 now precedes the H because the S_2 (V_2) impulse reaches the atria via AP while blocking in the HPS of NP. A linking by interference results in the LBB because the latter is last to be activated during the RV pacing. The process of linking continues even when the pacing is stopped because the impulse cannot engage the RB to produce a QRS complex. Further shortening of S_2S_2 to 290 milliseconds, (*panel C from top*) the initial linking is followed by forward migration and a QRS complex with an LBBB pattern (*asterisk*). The QRS occurs before the stimulus, which is ineffective as the primary stimulus, and an orthodromic tachycardia is initiated with linking in the LBB. Events in A and B are also shown schematically with corresponding designations (ie, *A–C*). The stippled area in schema C represents the first complex of the orthodromic tachycardia shown by the asterisk in C. (*Adapted from* Lehmann MH, Denker S, Mahmud R, et al. Linking: a dynamic electrophysiologic phenomenon in macroreentry circuit. Circulation 1985;71:260; with permission.)

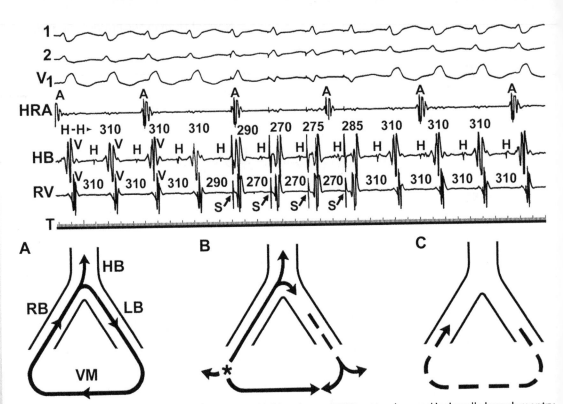

Fig. 23. Linking by collision. A ventricular tachycardia (showing an RBBB pattern) caused by bundle branch reentry (BBR) is shown. Note AV dissociation and a long HV of 100 milliseconds. The circuit of BBR VT is shown in A. When RV pacing at CL of 270 milliseconds is initiated, it enters the same path (ie, retrograde, into RBB; *B*) but also travels transseptally, colliding with anterograde impulse emerging from the LBB. The paced impulse reaches the HB and the QRS (resetting). The QRS activation is via 2 fronts and so is a fusion QRS complex (not fully paced or like tachycardia). This repeated appearance of QRS (entrainment with fusion) continues with collision of the paced impulse with the tachycardia impulse exiting from the LBB (linking by collision). As soon as the pacing is stopped, the tachycardia returns to its previous CL of 310 milliseconds. *, pacing site. (*From* Lehmann MH, Denker S, Mahmud R, et al. Linking: a dynamic electrophysiologic phenomenon in macro-reentry circuit. Circulation 1985;71:261; with permission.)

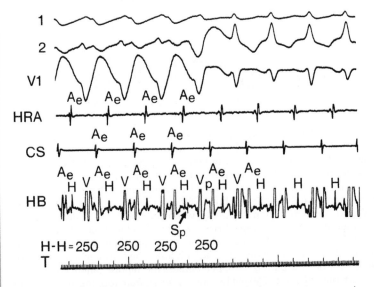

Fig. 24. Abolition functional BBB (demonstration of both types of linking phenomena). During an orthodromic AV reentry, the QRS shows a sustained LBBB, a single extrastimulus (S_p) is inducted after the HB potential is registered. There is no change in the H-H interval, but the QRS complex normalizes. The mechanism of loss of aberrancy includes both forms of linking, without which this phenomenon cannot be explained. The ventricular premature complex retrograde collides in some distal point of RBBB with oncoming anterograde reentrant impulse (linking by collision in the RBBB). Because the QRS shows LBBB during AV reentry, the right bundle impulse would otherwise have activated the ventricle. In the LBB, linking by interference has been going on during the tachycardia. The ventricular premature complex must break the link as well, which was by interference. However, the premature impulse can shorten LBBB-RP at the linking site if it can reach the linking site. If that happens, it may perpetuate the phenomenon. However, a more realistic possibility is that the premature ventricular impulse blocks more distal to the site of linking, which stops linking because of the lack of retrograde impulse penetration causing the anterograde impulse to move distal from the site of linking and reach the ventricle unless a distal site of linking is established. The terms to explain this phenomenon, such as peeling back of the RP, are not only vague but electrophysiologically inaccurate.

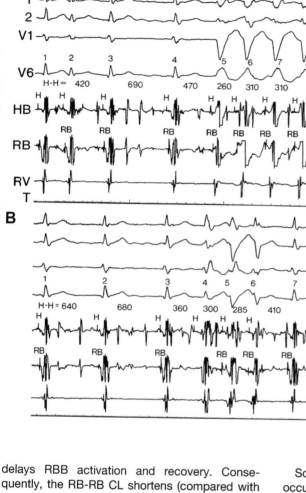

Fig. 25. Abolition of aberrant conduction. Any time a pause is created following an aberrantly conducted complex by a single or series of premature complexes functional aberrant conduction will abolish as long as the pause is sufficient to exceed the RP of a given BB or fascicle. During atrial fibrillation (A, B) a brief run of aberrancy disappears following the pause because of AV nodal delay. The pause can be created anywhere above the site of previous block. The numbers refer to individual QRS complexes and H-H values are in milliseconds.

delays RBB activation and recovery. Consequently, the RB-RB CL shortens (compared with the corresponding H-H-CL) and the next (A_2) conducts normally because of the abbreviation of RBB-RRP. When there is no RBBB, as occurs with the next A_2, RB-RB CL prolongs and the next A_2 shows conduction delay in the RBB. The first and the last A_2 conduct normally due to the absence of short-long-short sequence because the short-long-short sequence increases the RP of the HPS (see **Fig. 29**).[40] When the coupling interval of $A_1 A_2$ and consequently H_1H_2 is progressively shortened in a paced bigeminy model (see **Fig. 32**) there are a series of events that are noted, and these phenomena are common. Panel A shows that alternate A_2 conducts with either leftward axis and RBBB and left axis only. Further shortening of H-H CL (panel B) leads to RBBB with every A_2. In both panels the HV interval remains unchanged because the RP of the left posterior fascicles has not been reached. Panel C shows alternation of RBBB and LBBB, and the mechanisms of these occurrences are similar to what was discussed earlier and shown in **Fig. 30**.

Some other findings are worth mentioning: the occurrence of LBBB in panel C is not because the RP of the LBB exceeds that of the RB in this instance. The reason is concomitant H_2V_2 prolongation, which implies that RBB delay already exists (see **Fig. 10**B, C, and **Fig. 32**A, B). The site of delay in panel C is between H_2 and RB_2, because RB_2-V_2 interval equals the normal RB-V interval seen in the reference sinus complex (the last complex in panel D). Further shortening in H_1H_2 (panel D) results in all of A_2 encountering ERP of the HPS (no QRS) and the site of block is proximal (ie, H_2 no RB_2). The repetition of A_2 block in the HPS occurs because the H_2 impulse does not propagate beyond the site of H_2 block, so each impulse distal to the H_2 block site H_2 responds to a long HPS CL beyond the H_2 block site.

His-Purkinje System and Gap Phenomena

Another finding during extrastimulation is the so-called gap phenomenon. Simply put, it means that, at a given A_1A_2 coupling interval, A_2 blocks and there is no V_2 (**Figs. 33–35**).[5,43,44] At shorter

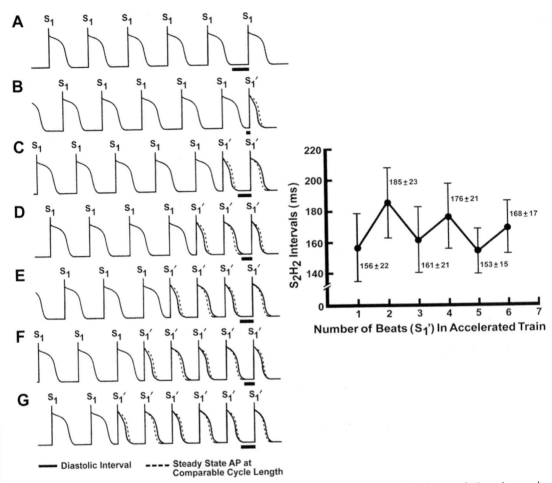

Fig. 26. Damped oscillation of HPS RP. (*A–G*) A specific ventricular pacing protocol is shown, designed to understand the effects of progressive shortening of the CL before the premature ventricular complex 1 to 6 shorter CLs (S'_1) before the premature complex S_2 (not shown in the pacing protocol). The steady state CL S_1 is shown before S'_1. Because the RP usually reflects the prior resting diastolic duration (the diastolic interval), it is shown as a solid black horizontal line under the diastolic interval for the last CL. The dotted action potential reflects the stead state action's potential duration at comparable CL. The number of $S'_1S'_1$ is progressively increased up to 6 S'_1. The results are shown on the right side of the panel where the number of S'_1 CL is plotted against the resulting S_2H_2 interval. The alternate S'_1 produces longer and shorter S_2H_2 intervals with a progressive decrease in the magnitude of S_2H_2 delay that parallels the diastolic interval shown. Such gradually damped behavior of the HPS can also be a mechanism of gradual shortening of HPS RP and eventual abolition of aberrant conduction. (*Adapted from* Tchou P, Lehmann MH, Dongas J, et al. Effect of sudden rate acceleration on the human His-Purkinje system: adaptation of refractoriness in a dampened oscillatory pattern. Circulation 1986;73:926–8; with permission.)

A_1A_2 the conduction resumes to the ventricles; an unexpected finding often interpreted as an example of supernormal conduction.[5] When this is seen with the help of HB recording, a simple event is noted to explain this observation. In so-called type I gap (there are several types), initially A_1A_2 blocks in HPS; that is, ERP of HPS is encountered at a certain H_1H_2 interval and exceeds that of the AVN and the AV impulse blocks below H_2 potential (see **Fig. 33**B). At shorter A_1A_2 coupling, the

A_2H_2 prolongs sufficiently such that the resultant H_1H_2 exceeds the ERP of HPS where the block was initially encountered (panel C). The H_1H_2 interval noted in panel C is therefore longer than in panel B and, because of this, conducts to V_2.[5,43] The disappearance of a BBB and/or H_2V_2 prolongation in a similar situation is a less dramatic form of type I gap. In type I gap the initial site of block and location of proximal delay are in different tissues (ie, the HPS and AVN,

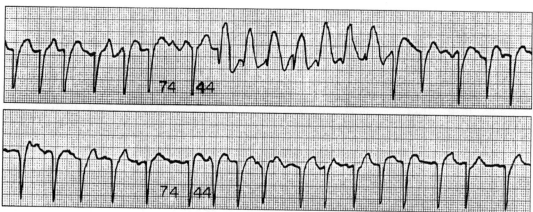

Fig. 27. Long-short CL sequence and aberrant conduction.[38,39] The surface ECG tracing (both panels) taken from Katz and colleagues[40] showing atrial fibrillation in the same patient. For the same long-short CL sequence (ie, 740 and 440 milliseconds, respectively), there is aberrant conduction in the top panel but not in the bottom. Concealed conduction in the HPS during the long cycle in the bottom panel was suggested as the explanation of unexpected shortening of the HPS refractoriness, which is different from the Ashman phenomenon.[38,39] This tracing and our own experience with rhythm strip analysis led us to design a pacing protocol (**Fig. 28**) that can simulate short-long, long-short, and various combinations in order to deduce the possible mechanism. (*From* Landgendorf R. Specific mechanisms of various disorders of impulse formation, conduction and their combinations. In: Langendorf R, Pick A, editors. Interpretation of Complex Arrhyhthmias. Philadelphia: Lea & Febiger (Springer);1979. p. 518; with permission.)

respectively). In type II gap (see **Fig. 34**), both sites are in the HPS.[43,44] **Fig. 34B** shows the infra-His block with resumption of conduction (panel C) where the H_1H_2 is even shorter. Slower conduction at a site in the HPS proximal to the initial site of block allows resumption of conduction. Note that the H_2V_2 and consequently V_1V_2 are longer in panel C than in panel A. Prolonged H_2V_2 may

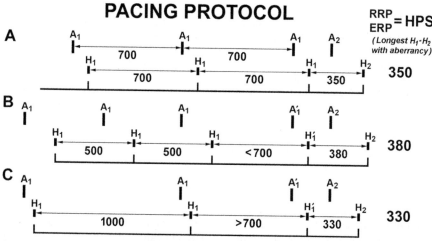

Fig. 28. Pacing protocol to study HPS response to long-short, short-long CL change.[40] (*A*) The reference stable atrial CL of 700 milliseconds (ie, A_1A_1). The stable CL of 700, 500, and 1000 milliseconds (only the first 1 or 2 stable CLs are shown). (*A*) No change is made in atrial paced CL; (*B*) there is 500 to 700 milliseconds change (short-long change, 500–700 milliseconds in B; and C 1000–700 milliseconds, long-short sequence). The last CL before the premature H'_1 is the reference CL and at the atrial level measures 700 milliseconds in all panels and then the premature atrial complex A_2. All of the H-H intervals are labeled and the corresponding RRP is shown under H_1H_2. During short to long change, $H_1H'_1$ measures less than A_1, A'_1 because of the change in AH when the CL changes, which is indicated by less than or greater than 700 milliseconds for the reference CL. (*B*) Compared with A the RRP of HPS is longer and the reverse takes place in C. (See **Fig. 29** for the tracing RRP and/or ERP.)

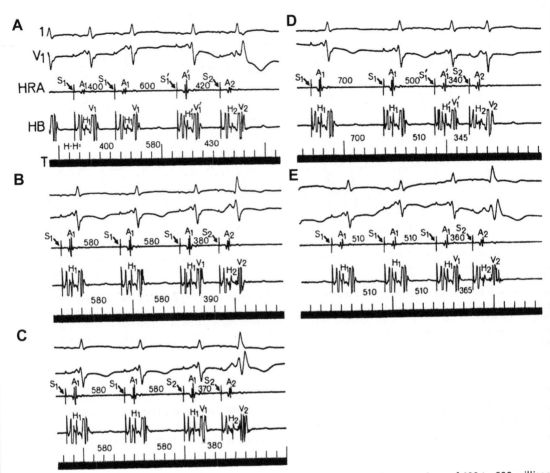

Fig. 29. Constant versus short to long/long to short CL change and HPS. (*A–C*) Comparison of 400 to 600 milliseconds atrial CL change after a series of constant 400 milliseconds (the last is shown). Because of the change from atrial pacing to 600 milliseconds the corresponding $H_1H'_1$ is 580 milliseconds. The results in A are compared with the results constant CL of 580 milliseconds (*B*). Note that the relative refractory period (RRP) of HPS (RBBB pattern) is increased by 50 milliseconds (430 vs 380 milliseconds). The opposite occurs when the CL is shortened (ie, L-S) in D compared with constant CL of 510 milliseconds (*E*). The $H_1H'_1$ adjustment from 500 to 510 milliseconds is for the same reason: $H_1H'_1$ increases with long to short CL change. In this case, RRP - HPS (RBBB) (*D, E*) shows more than a 20-millisecond decrease. (*Adapted from* Denker S, Shenasa M, Gilbert C, et al. Effects of abrupt changes in cycle length on refractoriness of the His-Purkinje system in man. Circulation 1983;67:64–5; with permission.)

reflect a bilateral or intra-His conduction delay even though no recordings along the BB were made. In type III gap the site of initial block and proximal delay are both within the HB (see **Fig. 35**).[45] Both proximal and distal sites of HPS block and eventual resumption of conduction with profound delay that can occur in normal HPS are shown in **Fig. 18**.

His-Purkinje System Response During Retrograde Propagation

The HPS physiologic phenomena are more commonly observed during the propagation of impulses in the retrograde direction, mainly because ventricular impulses encounter HPS first. The main limitation is the identification of retrograde HB activation, which is often obscured by the local ventricular electrogram, mostly during pacing with basic CL and late coupled extrastimuli (ie, >70% of the basic CL). The recognition of retrograde HB activation can be improved or its location determined by (1) using electrode catheters with a 1-mm to 2-mm interelectrode distance; (2) by simultaneously recording BB or fascicular electrograms; (3) by deducting the H_2A_2 interval from H_1V_1 after H_2 emergence; and (4) by the physiologic response of VA conduction in general, particularly the site of concealed conduction of the atrial rhythm (delay or block; ie, AVN vs HPS) during AV

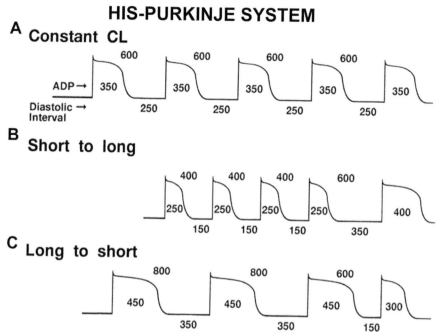

Fig. 30. Mechanisms of RRP-ERP HPS change with sudden CL change.[42] A possible explanation for the phenomena observed in **Fig. 29** and explained at a more basic cellular level. The constant CL APD of HPS and diastolic intervals are shown in A in milliseconds. If HPS response to diastolic interval rather than APD is accepted for HPS recovery, it becomes easier to explain the results seen in **Fig. 29**. The diastolic interval prolongs with a short to long change (*B*) and shortens with long to short change (*C*), so the corresponding RRP-HPS of HB and the magnitude of HPS-RP change could not be concluded from the APD. (*From* Akhtar M, Denker S, Lehmann M, et al. Effects of sudden cycle length alteration on refractoriness of human His-Purkinje system and ventricular myocardium. In: Zipes D, Jalife J, editors. Cardiac electrophysiology and arrhythmias. New York: Grune & Stratton Publishers; 1985. p. 406; with permission.)

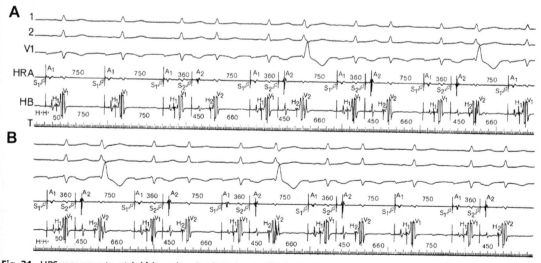

Fig. 31. HPS response to atrial bigeminy. During a controlled atrial bigeminy, by design the first 2 CLs in A and the last 2 CLs in B are kept constant at 750 milliseconds. Otherwise there is an atrial bigeminy where A_1A_2 measures 360 milliseconds and the next $A_2 A_1$ is 750 milliseconds, and this alternation continues (the 2 panels are not continuous). The corresponding H_2H_1 and H_1H_2 are labeled. See text for detailed explanation. (*From* Denker S, Lehmann MH, Mahmud R, et al. Effects of alternating cycle lengths on refractoriness of the His-Purkinje system in man. J Clin Invest 1984;74:561; with permission.)

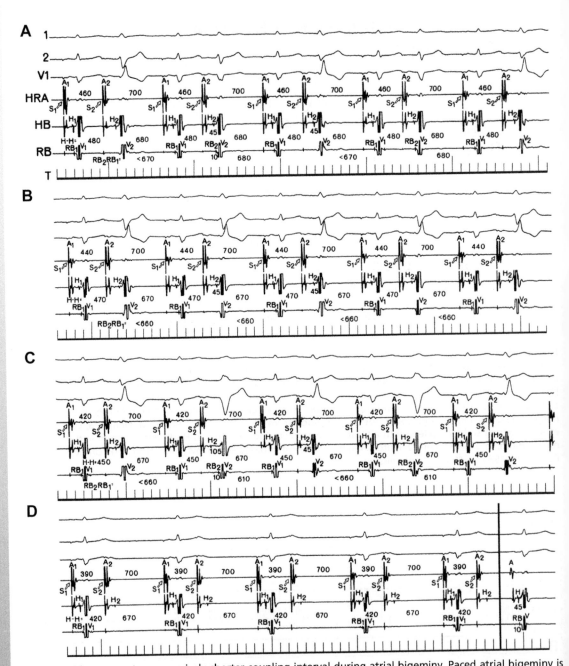

Fig. 32. HPS response to progressively shorter coupling interval during atrial bigeminy. Paced atrial bigeminy is seen in all 4 panels. The A_1A_2 is progressively shortened from A to D (ie, 460, 440, 420, and 390 milliseconds, respectively. The A_2A_1 interval is the same at 700 milliseconds in all panels. There is additional RB recording with RB-V interval of 20 milliseconds and H-RB of 35 milliseconds during sinus (the last complex in *D*) and all normal QRS complexes. The RB potential merges into local V electrogram before all QRS complexes showing an RBBB pattern; hence, the RB-RB interval now measures less than the H-H interval (shown with the symbol <). With progressive shortening of H_1H_2 a variety of HPS responses occur; namely, BB (both R and L), HV prolongation, and block below the His bundle (BBH). The site of delay and block is between H and RB. See text for details. (*From* Denker S, Lehmann MH, Mahmud R, et al. Effects of alternating cycle lengths on refractoriness of the His-Purkinje system in man. J Clin Invest 1984;74:564; with permission.)

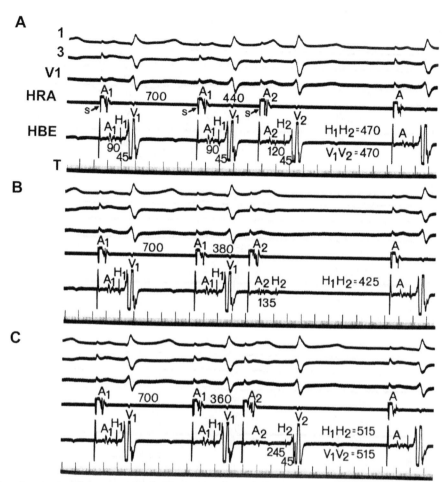

Fig. 33. Type I gap phenomenon (anterograde). At a basic atrial paced CL of 700 milliseconds, progressively shorter A_1A_2 are shown in A to C. At H_1H_2 of 470 milliseconds (*A*) AV nodal delay ($A_2 H_2$) is normal, and so are $H_2 V_2$ and QRS. At shorter A_1A_2, the H_1H_2 is 425 milliseconds (*B*), and the H2 impulse blocks in the HPS (H_2 but no V_2). At even shorter A_1A_2 at 360 milliseconds (*C*), the A_2 conducts to the QRS similar to A. The HB tracing shows the reason. The conduction delay $A_2 H_2$ (AVN) prolongs with resultant H_1H_2 to 515 milliseconds, which is outside the RRP and ERP of HPS so it conducts normally. At times, such an occurrence has been attributed to supernormal conduction, but proximal delay of conduction allows the site of such initial block to recover excitability (ie, H_1H_2 that conducts is longer than one that blocks). This phenomenon in essence is the reason (ie, proximal conduction delay and distal recovery) for all types of gap phenomenon. (*Adapted from* Gallagher JJ, Damato AN, Caracta AR, et al. Gap in A-V conduction in man. Types I and II. Am Heart J 1973;85:78–82 and Akhtar M, Damato AN, Batsford WP, et al. Unmasking and conversion of gap phenomenon in the human heart. Circulation 1974;49:627; with permission.)

dissociation. In patients with normal intraventricular conduction (NIVC) and/or intact retrograde RBB conduction, if the HB potential is recognizable during right ventricle (RV) pacing it will precede the local V electrogram (**Fig. 36A**)[16,26] or is buried in it. When there is conduction delay or block in BB ipsilateral to the pacing site the HB potential may be identifiable at the end of local V electrogram (see **Fig. 36B**). This situation is further discussed later in relation to abnormal HPS.

In patients with NIVC the retrograde HPS is almost always intact so the V_1H_1 interval remains constant with gradual shortening in the CL, as happens during anterograde HPS conduction (HV). At coupling interval (V_1V_2) less than 50% of basic CL or shorter than 300 milliseconds and with sudden onset of pacing, at least 4 responses may be observed.[46] One or more may be seen in the same individual, depending on (1) initial CL of pacing, (2) the coupling interval between the first and second train of stimuli, and (3) the CL of the second train (see **Figs. 6** and **14**).

Fig. 14 shows an example of 2 of these HPS responses using the pacing protocols, shown in

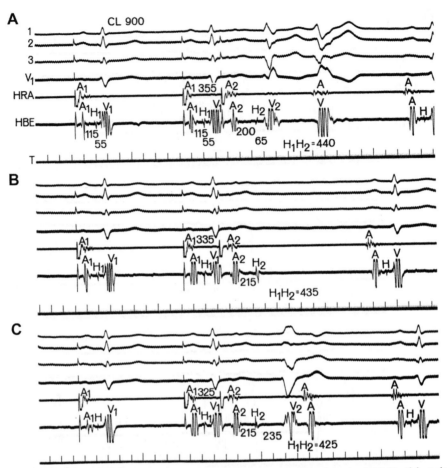

Fig. 34. Type II gap phenomenon (anterograde). Here the initial site of block is also HPS (*A, B*) but shorter A_1A_2 and H_1H_2 compared with **Fig. 33** conducts with a long HV and LBBB pattern (*C*). The sites of block and proximal delay permitting distal recovery of excitability are therefore both infra-Hisian. (*From Akhtar M, Sra JS. Physiological responses during electrophysiologic evaluation. In: Sra JS, Akhtar M, editors. Practical Electrophysiology. Minneapolis (MN): Cardiotext; 2014. p. 59; with permission.*)

Fig. 5C. The initial atrial train measures 500 milliseconds (panels A and B). Stimulus artifact (S_1) in the HV can be identified on the HB electrogram in the reference sinus complex (the last complex in panel A). There is a variable coupling interval (S_1S_2). Atrial pacing is depicted by a white arrow; ventricular pacing by a black arrow. The S_1S_2 (A_1V_2) coupling is 800 milliseconds and 400 milliseconds in panels A and B, respectively. All of the subsequent wide complexes labeled S_2 (V_2) are RV paced at a constant CL of 300 milliseconds. In panel A, the first 2 $S_2 S_2$ are short CL following a long couple interval, so the V_2H_2 delay is encountered in the HPS and the retrograde H_2 can be seen following the second V_2 and shortens to 150 milliseconds. This process is caused by linking by interference in the HPS. If the V_2 impulse reaches H_2 via the RB, the link will occur in LB and vice versa. Otherwise, a normal HPS does

not display this response of 1:1 VH conduction delay, which is constant but prolonged (ie, 1° anterograde or retrograde block HPS). There is concomitant H_2A_2 (AV nodal) Wenckebach (WP) that is subtle, and ends with H_2A_2 block (H_2 but no A_2) after 6th paced complex. The next 2 CLs show a 2:1 H_2A_2 block. By shortening of S_1S_2 coupling to 400 milliseconds (see **Fig. 14**B) there is no HPS delay despite the same paced CL of the second train of 300 milliseconds (ie, the H_2 has not emerged and remains obscured by the V_2 electrogram). However, the AVN (HA conduction) shows the same WP and 2:1 block as panel A. The S_2A_2 intervals are shorter in panel B because there is no HPS (VH) delay. Panel C is shown as a reference to confirm the H_2 emergence with a single V_2 during long-short VV CL, which is usually the rule rather than the exception. The second response in **Fig. 14**B is called

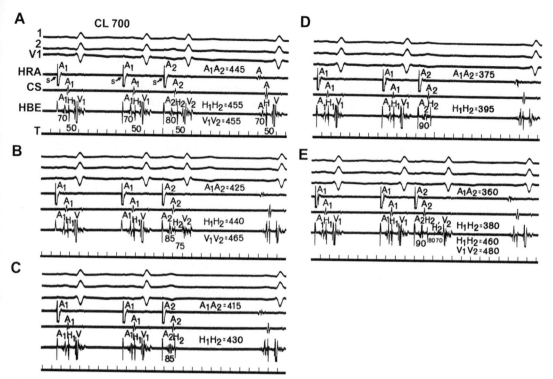

Fig. 35. Type III gap phenomenon (anterograde). The basic CL is 700 milliseconds, and A_1A_2 are progressively shortened (*A–E*). The A_2 impulse initially blocks in the HPS at H_1H_2 of 440 milliseconds and continues to block at H_1H_2 of 395 milliseconds (*D*). At even shorter H_1H_2, AV conduction revives with long HV, split His potential, and normal QRS. The sites of initial block and proximal delay are both in the HB. (*From* Damato AN, Akhtar M, Ruskin J, et al. Gap phenomena: anterograde and retrograde. In: Wellens HJJ, Lie KI, Janse MJ, editors. The conduction system of the heart. Philadelphia: Lea & Febiger (Springer); 1976. p. 512; with permission.)

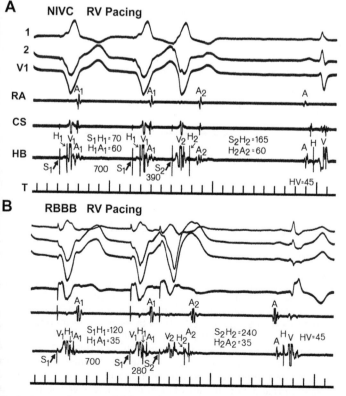

Fig. 36. HPS during retrograde conduction, showing retrograde H_1 location when it can be identified (*A* and *B* are from different patients). (*A*) The sinus rhythm shows normal intraventricular conduction (IVC) and HV interval of 45 milliseconds. During V_1V_1 retrograde H_1 is identifiable and precedes the local V_1 electrogram. Its rapid conduction and a brief duration suggest its HB potential, but this is confirmed with ventricular extrastimulus (V_2), which moves it to a location after V_2 electrogram. Now both V_2H_2 and H_2 A_2 can be clearly identified and measured. The early appearance of H_1 is because RV paced impulse reached the HB via RBB with no delay. The V_2 usually blocks in the retrograde RBB and H_2 activation occurs via the LBB after transseptal conduction. This pattern is the case in patients with V_1V_1 at baseline; that is, normal QRS and normal HV interval. The patient in B has a complete RBBB pattern during sinus rhythm. The HV is normal because of normal conduction through the LBB. During RV pacing (as in *A*) the H_1, appears at the end of the V_1 electrogram because of retrograde RBB and its activation via LBB, adding transseptal conduction time. With V_2 the H_2 moves farther away from V_2 electrogram because of delay in the LBB. Note that the S_1H_1 in B is 50 milliseconds longer than A (typical transseptal conduction) and both tracings show rapid H_2A_2 conduction (ie, $H_2A_2<60$ milliseconds).

accommodation, which continues indefinitely, whereas the linking phenomenon seen in panel A usually ends at a variable interval because of migration of the site of linking. See also **Fig. 22B** and C.

The third response is repetition of HPS WP or 2:1 block in the HPS for a variable period until accommodation with 1:1 stable VH conductions (**Fig. 37A** and C). The pattern of 3:2 or 2:1 may be followed by 1:1 conduction with a BBB because, like the anterograde counterpart, retrograde conduction recovers asynchronously regardless of the chamber of origin and the VH interval could abruptly shorten with disappearance of ipsilateral BBB (**Fig. 37C**) with impulse migration as the damped oscillatory behavior suggests. This process was referred to earlier, but is more relevant to mention here because it was studied

during retrograde propagation (see **Fig. 26**).[37] The fourth response is the migration of the linking phenomenon or site of block until the impulse reaches the HB via the ipsilateral BB without conduction delay. Any of the impulse that reaches the HB is likely to penetrate the AVN with a variety of responses. Because the AVN is not part of this communication, it is not detailed here unless relevant to the main topic (ie, the HPS). Similar to HPS behavior in an anterograde direction, patients with NIVC show no conduction delays in the HPS at constant long CL (ie, >500 milliseconds) and progressive and gradual rate acceleration. The responses to sudden bursts of shorter CL were outlined earlier with the exception of 1. At an extremely rapid rate (ie, a CL of $\leq$250 milliseconds), ventricular fibrillation can be induced even in patients with NIVC, and clinicians should be

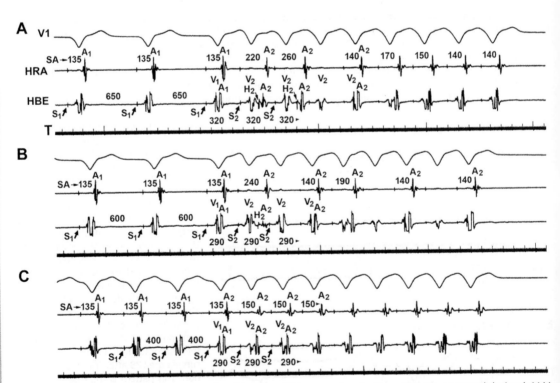

Fig. 37. The effect of variable basic CL and rapid and variable secondary train on HPS. The protocol design is V_1V_1 greater than V_2V_2 train (see **Fig. 5C**). The basic CL is 650 milliseconds in A, 600 milliseconds in B, and 400 milliseconds in C. The second train CL is 320 milliseconds in A and 290 milliseconds in B and C. The VA (S_1A_1) is 140 to 150 milliseconds in all panels as the baseline interval. With the onset of V pacing at 320 milliseconds (S_2S_2) in A, initially there is an HPS WP (4:3); that is, normal HPS (first S_1) prolonged S_2H_2 with second S_2 even longer S_2H_2 with the third S_2 and fourth S_2 blocks HPS (no H, no A). Subsequently, aside from a slight delay (to 170 milliseconds) with S_2 there is stable VA conduction to 140 milliseconds in B and there is initially a 3:2 HPS for 2 cycles and then 2:1 HPS block. (C) A rapid stabilization of VA to 150 milliseconds occurs because of shortening of S_1S_1 CL to 400 milliseconds. (A) Accommodation of the HPS; however, how this occurs depends on basic CL coupling interval, and the CL duration of the next train. The A_2A_2 is short and is not the site of delay or block with any of the paced impulses.

aware of this. In contrast, sustained monomorphic VT cannot be induced in normal individuals.

During scanning of the basic CL with progressively shorter $V_1 V_2$, some of the same phenomena are noted, as seen during anterograde conduction. During basic CL ventricular pacing, recognition of retrograde H_1 is difficult unless it precedes or follows the local V_1 electrogram (see **Fig. 36**). Even in those cases in which H_1 is identifiable, anterograde HPS (ie, $H_1 V_1$) and retrograde ($V_1 H_1$) conduction interval comparison is not precise. The 2 obvious reasons are that $V_1 H_1$ is usually measured from stimulus artifact (S_1), and almost always exceeds $H_1 V_1$ interval in the same patient. It is not clear how much of retrograde $S_1 H_1$ includes myocardial Purkinje conduction times. Retrograde $S_1 H_1$ as measured from stimulus artifact to onset of HB deflection

is not similar to $H_1 V_1$, because the latter is traditionally calculated from the onset of H_1 instead of its end, which is more comparable with retrograde $S_1 H_1$. When it is important to have this information, clinicians can attain it by multiple HPS recordings. Based on the measurement of such recordings, when available, it seems that conduction time in the HPS is similar in the 2 directions (**Fig. 38**).

The study of HPS during extrastimulation (V_2) reveals several other phenomena as well. Starting with the late ventricular extrastimulus ($V_1 V_2$) defined as greater than or equal to 70% of the basic CL, there is little or no conduction delay. If there is prolongation of $V_2 A_2$ compared with $V_1 A_1$ it is likely caused by increase in $H_2 A_2$ (AV nodal) conduction time (**Fig. 39**). Often a ventricular echo phenomenon caused by AV nodal reentry

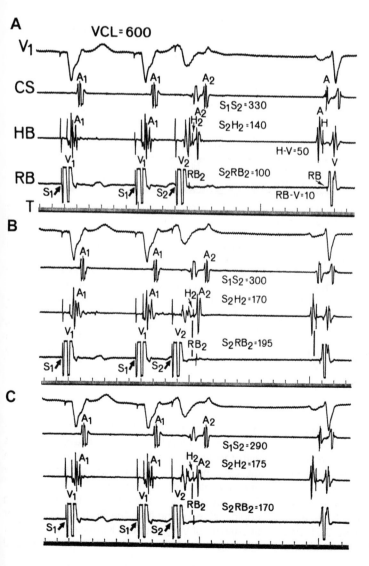

Fig. 38. Comparison of anterograde and retrograde HPS conduction. During ventricular pacing at a basic CL of 600 milliseconds, $S_1 S_2$ ($V_1 V_2$) intervals are reduced from 330 to 300 to 290 milliseconds (A–C). Although the retrograde H is identifiable, it is not labeled. The S_2 conducts to H_2 via RBB (RB$_2$). The RB$_2$-H$_2$ (40 milliseconds) measures exactly the same at anterograde H-RB of 40 milliseconds during sinus rhythm. The activation route to the HB changes in B, in which the H_2 now precedes RB$_2$ (H$_2$RB$_2$ 25 milliseconds) typical of HB activation via the LB. The reason is that, when the V_2 impulse arrives at the HB bifurcation site, it conducts retrograde toward the H_2 and anterograde toward the RB$_2$. Depending on the location of the H-RB recording electrode, H$_2$-RB$_2$ can be zero to a short HRB interval or equal to HRB of sinus. Note that the H_2 and RB$_2$ are activated at the same time in C, which can only happen if H_2 was activated via the LBB and RB$_2$ through the RBB. This conclusion is based on the HRB sequence in A and B and the reference sinus rhythm (the last complexes in all panels).

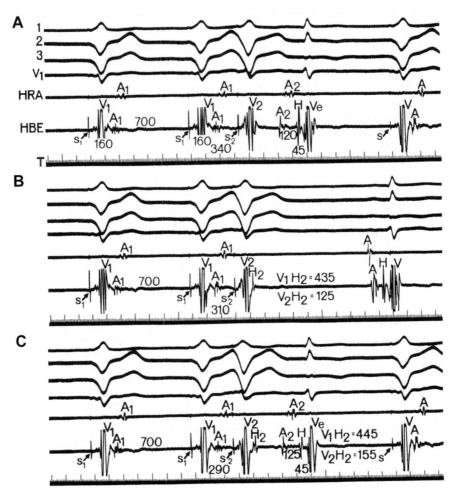

Fig. 39. HPS delays and recovery of AVN conduction. At a basic CL of 700 milliseconds, V_2 conducts with long V_2A_2 even before the H_2 emerges from V_2. The activation sequence of A_2 is low to high (the A_2 on HB precedes A_2 on HRA). It is followed by another activation of the HB, followed by a narrow QRS. This pattern is a classic example of so-called ventricular echo phenomenon (Ve) caused by AV nodal reentry. At a shorter coupling interval of 310 milliseconds (*B*) the H_2 emerges and the impulse blocks in the AVN (ie, no A_2) and AV nodal reentry is abolished. With further S_1S_2 shortening (*C*) the retrograde A_2 reemerges and is followed by the reappearance of ventricular echo phenomenon (retrograde type I gap). The reason is that now the retrograde H_1H_2 is longer in C than in B. However, because retrograde H_1 is not identifiable, V_1H_2 can be compared in the two panels. We have routinely used S_1-H_2 (V_1H_2) as a surrogate for H_1H_2 because S_1H_1 always has a constant value in patients with normal IVC and V_1 H_2 exceeds H_1H_2 by the same amount in all panels. The latter can be measured when the H_2 emerges. Note that the V_1H_2 in C is greater than in B. It is also worth noting that in response to V_2, in AV nodal reentry the HB must be activated twice: once in retrograde and then in the anterograde direction. Panels A and C both have double H_2 activations but it is clearly measureable in C.

follows (see **Fig. 39**). Once the retrograde H_2 emerges from V_2 electrogram S_2H_2 can be accurately measured. At this point S_2H_2 can be separated from H_2A_2 conduction times. Because the AVN responds to coupling of retrograde H_1H_2, not V_1V_2, if there is H_2A_2 delay needed for comparison it is better to use retrograde S_1H_2 as a surrogate for retrograde H_1H_2 because S_1H_1 has a constant value and retrograde H_1 is not always

visible. The moment the H_2 emerges from V_2 electrograms, it usually (but not always) coincides with the onset of retrograde block of S_2 (V_2) in the RB, and the V_2 impulse travels transseptally and activates the H_2 via the LBB (**Fig. 40**).[8,16] This process can be readily confirmed with an additional recording from the BB (**Fig. 41**). Further shortening of V_1V_2 coupling increases V_2H_2 delay, allowing the RBB to recover excitability and

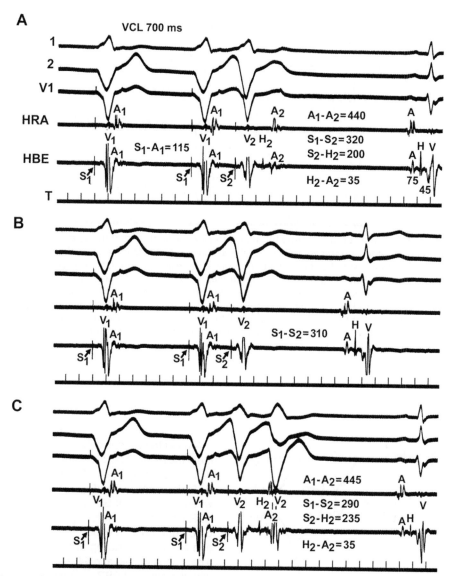

Fig. 40. Retrograde HPS conduction delay, block, reentry, and gap HPS. At 700-millisecond V_1V_1 the V_2 is delivered at V_1V_2 of 320 milliseconds (*A*), the retrograde H_2 emerges because it is activated via the LBB (this is clearer in *C*). At shorter S_1S_2 (*B*) V_2 blocks in the HPS (no H_2 or A_2). With further shortening of V_1V_2 the H_2 reemerges with longer V_2H_2 compared with A (retrograde type II gap). Note also that a spontaneous QRS follows that mimics V_2 in terms of QRS morphology axis with H_2V_3 interval longer than sinus. This pattern is a result of anterograde propagation through the RBB, which does not happen in A because of insufficient delay for RBB recovery. This V_3 phenomenon is caused by so-called BBR (discussed later), but confirms that H_2 was activated via the LBB in A as well.

effective propagation of the impulse along the RB, which results in a spontaneous QRS (V_3 phenomenon) showing LBBB pattern (see **Fig. 41**; **Fig. 42**).[16] This so-called reentry HPS (more commonly referred to as BBR)[12] is a purely physiologic phenomenon and is seen in approximately 50% of patients with NIVC. The morphology and axis of BBR suggest that it travels the same route as V_2, and it changes as the V_1V_2, V_2V_3 interval relationship changes. Reversal of BB activation sequence may occasionally produce BBR with an RBBB pattern despite RV pacing (**Fig. 43**). BBR usually occurs as a single complex that blocks retrograde in the HPS (ie, no H_3) and the process self-terminates (see **Figs. 41** and **43**).

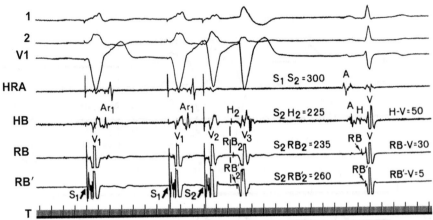

Fig. 41. BBR (Re HPS – bundle branch reentry [BBR]). During RV pacing note that the V_2 at a V_1V_2 of 300 milliseconds is followed by another spontaneous QRS complex similar to V_2. The 3 recordings along the H-RB axis, HB, proximal and distal RBB measure 50, 30, and 5 milliseconds, respectively, during sinus rhythm. Remarkably, the HRB sequence before V_3 is similar to sinus (ie, anterograde), whereas the RV is the pacing site. The only logical explanation is that the H_2 is activated via the LBB (H_2 to proximal RB_2 measures 10 milliseconds, which is 10 milliseconds shorter than sinus) but proximal RB_2 to distal RB_2 is 25 milliseconds, the same as sinus complex. This finding is a classic example of BBR with LBBB pattern when pacing RV. V_3 in turn blocks retrograde in HPS (no H_3) and the process terminates spontaneously. The sequence of HRB deflection suggests H_2 activation via the LBB as the only logical explanation.

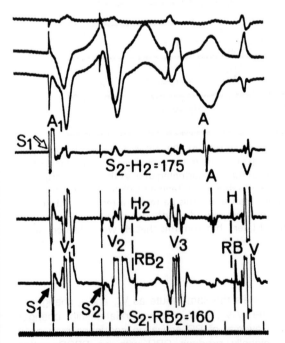

Fig. 42. BBR with RBBB pattern. The sequence of HPS activation is H>RB>QRS during sinus complex (the last complex in the tracing) and is reversed to RB–HV with BBR showing an RBBB and left axis deviation pattern even though the site of pacing is RV apex.

Among the various criteria used to initially document the nature of BBR, 1 stood out. Whenever the V_2 blocks retrograde in the HPS LBB (ie, no H_3), BBR does not occur (**Figs. 44** and **45**).[16] Rarely, when there is H_3, it blocks anterograde (ie, no V_4). BBR also stops if there is block in the RBB retrograde gap phenomenon. Return of V_2H_2 conduction at shorter coupling intervals (retrograde type II gap; see **Figs. 40** and **44**) and is often associated with the return of BBR.[42–46] It has been known for some time that a single ventricular premature complex (V_2) in the setting of ventricular pacing can produce 2 types of reentry: AV nodal and HPS. AV nodal reentry following V_2 requires activation of the HB twice (ie, once in the retrograde and then in the anterograde direction; **Fig. 45**),[25,26] whereas BBR needs activation of HB only once (see **Fig. 45**). Occasionally the 2 forms of echo (reentry) phenomenon coexist (**Fig. 46**).[47]

Although BBR per se is a physiologic event with no prognostic significance, the lack of its recognition may cause confusion about some electrophysiologic events. Some examples of these misinterpretations are as follows:

1. BBR is not common in the setting of sinus rhythm, but may occur if there is prolonged H-H CL (**Fig. 47**) preceding a spontaneous or

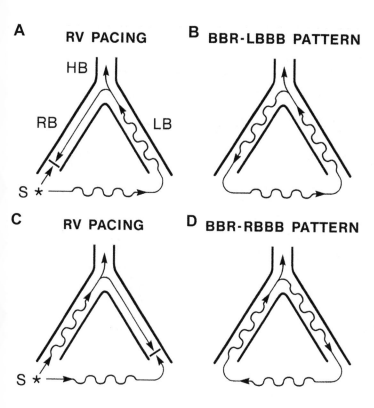

A   RV PACING   **B**   BBR-LBBB PATTERN

C   RV PACING   **D**   BBR-RBBB PATTERN

Fig. 43. Induction of BBR. The RV pacing site and retrograde block in RBB or LBB to initiate the process. With RV pacing, a premature complex is more likely to block retrograde in RBB causing the BBR to have an LBBB pattern. In the rare event that V_2 blocks in the LBB instead and reaches H2 via RBB, the sequence is reversed (ie, RB>H>V for BB R with an RBBB). *, stimulation site(s).

paced event, such as an implanted pacemaker. Although previously a ventricular couplet was given a prognostic significance in certain settings, it is obvious from **Fig. 47** that it is a benign event and that the 2 complexes even have different mechanisms. Not exactly comparable with the examples given earlier, the coexistence of 2 forms of ventricular echo phenomenon can also be taken as a prognostically serious event, but it is also benign (see **Fig. 46**).

2. In the setting of overt preexcitation and atrial tachycardias, such as atrial fibrillation, BBR may occur with different morphology (ie, depending on 1 or more of the AP locations) and make the ECG interpretation difficult.

3. An article from a prestigious institution published by a leading journal implied that a spontaneous V_3 following a V_2 identifies a high-risk population for sudden cardiac death.[48] The response of the literary academic electrophysiology community is discussed in Refs.[49–52]

Before ending the description of some of the HPS phenomena, a word of caution is needed. This article only covers the responses to single ventricular premature complex or a run of rapid pacing in patients with NIVC. These short runs of repetitive responses have no predictive significance even in patients with known VT.[50,51] It is

equally critical to realize that, during the conduct of these studies, extreme caution is used and latency between the stimulus artifact and local V response during multiple premature beats is avoided because even normal people can develop ventricular fibrillation. This condition occurs in patients with poor left ventricular function and has been shown previously.[53]

When conduction and retrograde RP curves are plotted, a frequently unique phenomenon is often observed in patients with rapid H-A conduction time, defined here as less than or equal to 60 milliseconds measured from the onset of H deflection to the onset of A deflection on the HB electrogram (during both H_1-A_1 and H_2 A_2). Throughout the scanning with progressively shorter V_1 V_2 intervals there appears to be no change in H_2 A_2 interval (**Fig. 48**).[54] The primary reason for this is that a V_1V_2 decrease almost equals a V_2H_2 increase, so the AV nodal input is no earlier; the V_1H_2 interval remains the same even though the V_1V_2 interval progressively shortens (see **Fig. 48**).[54] Sometimes this has been equated to a behavior of the AV nodal bypass tract. If the retrograde H_1 H_2 interval can somehow be shortened (eg, with a shorter basic CL), then H_2 A_2 interval prolongation will be noted as well as with pharmacologic agents that traditionally suppress AV nodal conduction

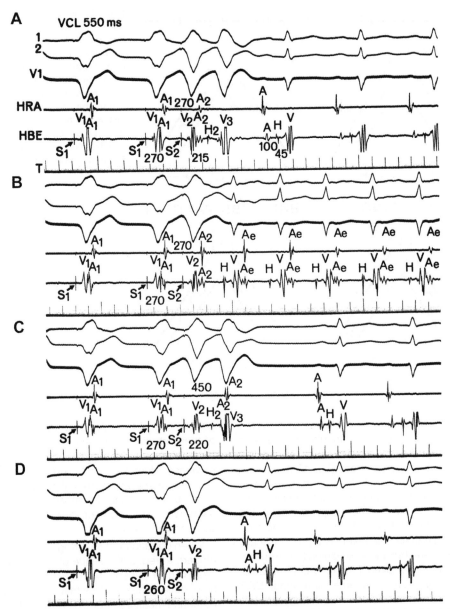

Fig. 44. Relationship of HPS and BBR and onset of AV reentry. In a patient with concealed right-sided AP, basic CL 550 milliseconds with V_1V_2 of 270 milliseconds (A–C) V_1V_2 is 260 milliseconds (D). Retrograde conduction via AP is immediately noticeable because A_2 in A precedes the H_2 activation. The V_2 also activates retrograde H_2 via the LBB and is followed by V_3 (BBR), which does not activate H_3 or A_3 via any pathway. The next time (B) V_2 blocks in the HPS and produces A_2 via the AP. Now the A_2 finds AVN recovered excitability (not penetrated by V_2 because of block in the HPS) conducts through AVN-HPS and initiates the AV reentry (orthodromic). Incidentally, this is the most common mechanism of orthodromic SVT conduction during RV pacing (extrastimulus or constant CL pacing). The $A_2 H_2$ is shorter than the subsequent AH intervals supporting V_2 block in the HPS. The third time, the V_2 blocks in the AP and conducts to the atria via the AVN (ie, H_2 precedes A_2). There is the return of BBR, suggesting that activation of H_2 is critical for the occurrence of BBR. At V_1V_2 of 260 milliseconds (D) V_2 blocks along both (ie, in the HPS and AP so there is no BBR or orthodromic SVT). V_2 responses of HPS (A–C) also are examples of retrograde type II gap phenomenon in the HPS. The elaborate $V_2 H_2$ conduction and BBR (A) V_2H_2 block and SVT (B) $V_2 H_2$ conduction and BBR but no SVT. Findings in (C) also illustrate why orthodromic AVR is not initiated 1) V_3 did not produce A_3 via the accessory pathway and 2) even if that had occurred, the AV node will be difficult to negotiate by A_3 due to prior invasion of retrograde H_2 impulse.

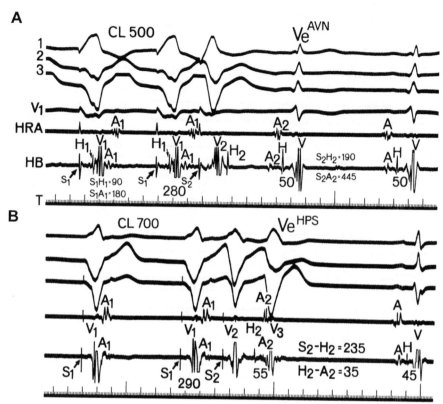

Fig. 45. Two types of ventricular echo phenomenon with V_2. The nature of the 2 forms of ventricular echo phenomenon is labeled. The key difference is that the HB is activated twice before Ve AVN (ie, *A* shows a narrow QRS) and only once in B (Ve HPS) and a wide QRS.

(ie, β-blockers and calcium channel blockers). Occasionally, with proper timing, H_2A_2 block may be induced with carotid sinus massage (CSM) (**Fig. 49**).[54] The observations mentioned earlier are generally noted in 20% to 30% of the population. The reason this type of AV nodal behavior is covered here is because the HPS delays (ie, retrograde H_1H_2 [V_1H_2]) are responsible for this type of AV nodal response and are not caused by the presence of the AV nodal bypass tract (see **Figs. 40** and **41**). The other individuals have either longer HA (see **Figs. 39**, **45**, and **46**)[8] or no HA conduction (**Fig. 50**); that is, unidirectional block, which is often functional and can be reversed (see **Fig. 50**).[55] In these patients, other rules of AV nodal behavior also apply. All of this is explainable from V_1H_2; when this is within the AV nodal ERP there is a block, and if it is outside the ERP, the conduction resumes (retrograde type I gap; see **Fig. 39**).[45]

SUMMARY

Although many of the functional and/or physiologic aspects of HPS are covered, the key messages in this article are:

1. LBB has 3 divisions and evidence is presented with emphasis that the septal division is functional both in the anterograde and retrograde directions.

2. In individuals with normal baseline HPS, all of the phenomena (ie, BBB, HV prolongation, and complete block in the HPS) are normal events.

3. Many of the physiologic properties of the HPS (ie, conduction, RP) are similar in anterograde and retrograde directions.

4. A thorough study of the HPS requires additional recordings from the BB or fascicles. The lack of at least 1 additional recording from the RB or LB can lead to misinterpretation, especially when the APs are also involved. This statement is based on examples in published literature.

5. Whether some of the details here are necessary for good patient care may be debatable. However, knowledge of these concepts is important to understand and meet the minimal teaching standards of electrophysiology for a good foundation.

6. For progress in medicine in any discipline, it is essential to keep asking questions. If the

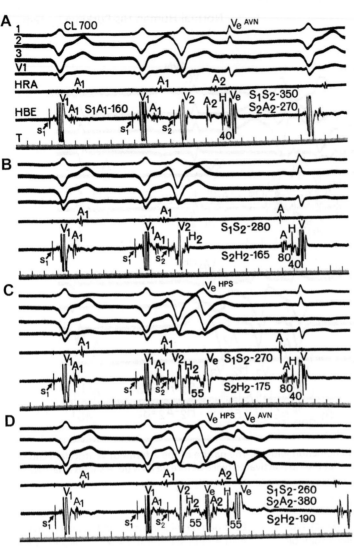

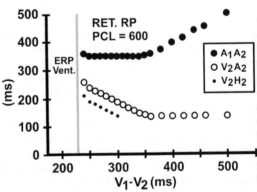

Fig. 48. Retrograde HPS delay and AVN response. In patients with short H_2A_2 (or H_1A_1; ie, ≤60 milliseconds) the H_2A_2 does not seem to increase with progressive decrease of the V_1V_2 intervals, which are plotted against V_2H_2, V_2A_2 and A_1A_2. Once the H_2 emerges, the H_2A_2 can be measured. Note the parallel relationship between H_2 and A_2. The reason for this constancy is that the V_2H_2 increase is about equal to V_1V_2 decrease, so that the retrograde impulse reaching the AVN (ie, V_1H_2) remains the same, so there is no change in H_2A_2. This fixed interval is not a reflection of an AV nodal bypass tract. PCL, pacing cycle length; RET-RP, retrograde refractory period.

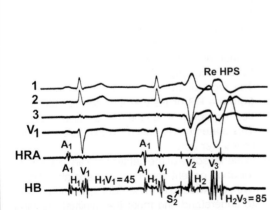

Fig. 47. BBR during sinus rhythm. Although unusual, BBR can occur following a single ventricular extrastimulus during sinus rhythm. The reason for its infrequency in patients with NIVC is that diverging wave fronts (ie, V pacing during sinus) cannot produce a sufficient delay in the HPS to produce BBR.

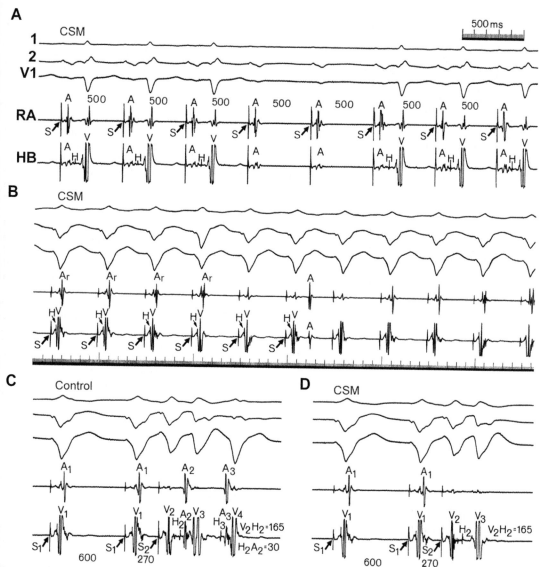

Fig. 49. Short H_2A_2 (AVN or AV nodal bypass tract) in a patient with short H_2A_2 of 30 milliseconds (*C*). The H_2 is followed by BBR and A_2 conducts anterograde to the ventricle via the AVN and is aberrant because of interposing BBR. CSM is known to suppress AV nodal conduction (ie, anterograde AV nodal block [*A*] and retrograde HA block during constant CL pacing [*B*]), and H_2A_2 conduction block abolishes AVN reentry (last complex in C) (*D*). The same pathway can be blocked with β-blockers and calcium channel blockers like much of AV nodal behavior. (*Adapted from* Akhtar M. Supraventricular tachycardias: electrophysiologic mechanisms, diagnosis and pharmacologic therapy. In: Josephson ME, Wellens HJJ, editors. Tachycardias: mechanisms, diagnosis and treatment. Philadelphia: Lea and Febiger (Springer); 1984:150–1; with permission.)

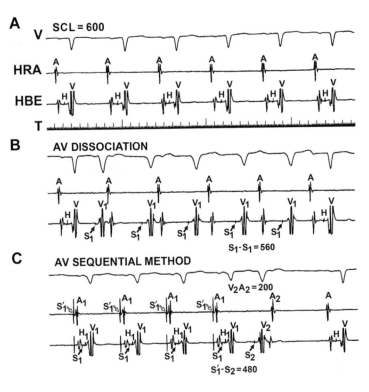

Fig. 50. Physiologic nature of no ventriculoatrial conduction. Sinus rhythm with normal PR, QRS, AH, and HV(*A*). At a CL of 560 milliseconds, just shorter than sinus (600 milliseconds), ventricular pacing is initiated (S_1S_1) and AV dissociation is observed (*B*). Despite increasing the V to A relationship, there is no AV conduction until the pacing is stopped (*B*). Penetration of the AVN by nonconducting V_1V_1 makes it difficult to conduct. This phenomenon is an example of linking by interference and the site is the AVN. Alternatively, AV dissociation is caused by concealed penetration of the AVN, which can be appreciated by conduction delay and block of dissociated sinus complex when the interference is prevented by AV sequential pacing (*C*). Now the V_2 is not interfered with by A and able to conduct and produce a retrograde atrial activated V_2A_2 interval of 200 milliseconds. (*Adapted from* Mahmud R, Denker S, Lehmann MH, et al. The effect of AV sequential pacing in patients with no ventriculoatrial conduction. J Am Coll Cardiol 1984;4:276; with permission.)

answer is not known, it can be learned with some investigative work.

7. In addition, this article is somewhat biased toward challenging the concepts rather than accepting any concept not proven to readers satisfaction.

ACKNOWLEDGMENTS

The author would like to acknowledge his appreciation for the tremendous support that he received in preparation of this article from Laurel Landis, Susan Nord, Jennifer Pfaff, and Brian Miller.

REFERENCES

1. Scherlag BJ, Lau SH, Helfant RH, et al. Catheter technique for recording His bundle activity in man. Circulation 1969;39:13–8.

2. Damato AN, Lau SH, Helfant RH, et al. A study of heart block in man using His bundle recording. Circulation 1969;39:297–305.

3. Narula OS, Scherlag BJ, Samet P, et al. Atrioventricular block. Localization and classification by His bundle recordings. Am J Med 1971;50:146–65.

4. Gallagher JJ, Damato AN, Caracta AR, et al. Gap in A-V conduction in man. Types I and II. Am Heart J 1973;85:78–82.

5. Damato AN, Varghese PJ, Caracta AR, et al. Functional 2:1 AV block within the His-Purkinje system: simulation of type II second degree AV block. Circulation 1973;47:534–42.

6. Coumel PH, Attuel P. Reciprocating tachycardia in overt and latent preexcitation: influence of functional bundle branch block on the rate of the tachycardia. Eur J Cardiol 1974;1:423–36.

7. Wellens HJJ, Durrer D. The role of an accessory atrioventricular pathway in reciprocal tachycardia. Observations in patients with and without the Wolff-Parkinson-White syndrome. Circulation 1975;52:58–72.

8. Akhtar M, Gilbert CJ, Al-Nouri M, et al. Site of conduction delay during functional block in the His-Purkinje system in man. Circulation 1980;61:1239–48.

9. Akhtar M. Atrioventricular nodal reentry. Circulation 1987;75:III26–30.

10. Josephson ME, editor. Clinical cardiac electrophysiology: techniques and interpretations. 4th edition. Philadelphia: Lippincott Williams & Wilkins; 2008.

11. Akhtar M, Damato AN, Caracta AR, et al. Electrophysiologic effect of atropine on atrioventricular conduction studied by His bundle electrogram. Am J Cardiol 1974;33:333–43.

12. Wellens HJJ, Lie KL, Durrer D. Further observations on ventricular tachycardia as studied by electrical stimulation of the heart. Chronic recurrent ventricular tachycardia and ventricular tachycardia during acute myocardial infarction. Circulation 1974;49: 647–53.

13. Akhtar M, Damato AN, Ruskin JN, et al. Anterograde and retrograde conduction characteristics in three patterns of paroxysmal atrioventricular junctional reentrant tachycardia. Am Heart J 1978;95:22–42.

14. Josephson ME, Kastor JA. His-Purkinje conduction during retrograde stress. J Clin Invest 1978;61: 171–7.

15. Akhtar M, Damato AN, Batsford WP, et al. Demonstration of re-entry within the His-Purkinje system in man. Circulation 1974;50:1150–62.

16. Akhtar M, Damato AN, Batsford WP, et al. A comparative analysis of anterograde and retrograde conduction patters in man. Circulation 1975; 52:766–78.

17. Narula OS. Retrograde preexcitation. Comparison of anterograde and retrograde conduction intervals in man. Circulation 1974;50:1129–43.

18. Reddy CP, Slack JD. Recurrent sustained ventricular tachycardia: report of a case with His-bundle branches reentry as the mechanism. Eur J Cardiol 1980;11:23–31.

19. Willhelm His Jr, MD. 1863-1934.

20. Jan Evangelista Purkinje. 1787-1869.

21. Kulbertus HD, Demoulin JCL. Pathological basis of concept of left hemiblock. In: Wellens HJJ, Lie KI, Janse MJ, editors. The conduction system of the heart: structure, function and clinical implications. New York: Springer; 1978. p. 287–95.

22. Hecht HH, Kossmann CE, Childers RW, et al. Atrioventricular and intraventricular conduction-revised nomenclature and concepts. Am J Cardiol 1973; 31:232–44.

23. Dhala A, Gonzalez-Buelgaray J, Deshpande S, et al. Unmasking the trifascicular left intraventricular conduction system by ablation of the right bundle branch. Am J Cardiol 1996;77:706–12.

24. Sung RK, Kim AM, Tseng ZH, et al. Diagnosis and ablation of multiform fascicular tachycardia. J Cardiovasc Electrophysiol 2013;24:297–304.

25. Durrer D, Schoo L, Schuilenburg RM, et al. The role of premature beats in the initiation and termination of supraventricular tachycardia in the Wolff-Parkinson-White syndrome. Circulation 1967;36:644–62.

26. Akhtar M, Mahmud R, Tchou PJ, et al. Normal electrophysiologic responses of the human heart. In: Horowitz LH, editor. Cardiology clinics of North America. Philadelphia: WB Saunders; 1986. p. 365–86.

27. Akhtar M, Sra JS. Physiological responses during electrophysiologic evaluation. In: Sra JS, Akhtar M, editors. Practical electrophysiology. Minneapolis (MN): Cardiotext; 2014. p. 39–108.

28. Akhtar M, Lehmann MH, Denker S, et al. Role of His Purkinje system in the initiation of orthodromic tachycardia in Wolff-Parkinson White syndrome. In: Benditt DG, Benson DW, editors. Cardiac Preexcitation syndromes. New York: Martinus Nijhoff Publishing (Springer); 1986. p. 141–50.

29. Denker S, Gilbert CJ, Shenasa M, et al. An electrocardiographic-electrophysiologic correlation of aberrant ventricular conduction in man. J Electrocardiol 1983;16:269–77.

30. Denker S, Lehmann MH, Mahmud R, et al. Effects of alternating cycle lengths on refractoriness of the His-Purkinje system in man. J Clin Invest 1984;74:559–70.

31. Akhtar M, Lehmann MH, Denker ST, et al. Electrophysiologic mechanisms of orthodromic tachycardia initiation during ventricular pacing in the Wolff-Parkinson-White syndrome. J Am Coll Cardiol 1987;9: 89–100.

32. Jazayeri M, Caceres J, Tchou P, et al. Electrophysiologic characteristics of sudden QRS axis deviation during orthodromic tachycardia: role of functional fascicular block in localization of accessory pathway. J Clin Invest 1989;83:952–9.

33. Lehman MH, Tchou P, Mahmud R, et al. Electrophysiologic determinant of antidromic reentry induced during atrial extrastimulation: insights from a pacing model of the Wolff-Parkinson-White syndrome. Circ Res 1989;65:295–306.

34. Lehmann MH, Denker S, Mahmud R, et al. Linking: a dynamic electrophysiologic phenomenon in macroreentry circuit. Circulation 1985;71:254–65.

35. Jazayeri M, Sra J, Akhtar M. Wide QRS complexes: electrophysiology basis of a common electrocardiographic diagnosis. J Cardiovasc Electrophysiol 1992;3:365–93.

36. Akhtar M, Jazayeri M, Avitall B, et al. Electrophysiologic spectrum of wide QRS complex tachycardia. In: Zipes P, Jalife J, editors. Cardiac electrophysiology: from cell to bedside. Orlando (FL): WB Saunders; 1990. p. 635–46.

37. Tchou P, Lehmann MH, Dongas J, et al. Effect of sudden rate acceleration on the human His-Purkinje system: adaptation of refractoriness in a dampened oscillatory pattern. Circulation 1986;73: 920–9.

38. Myerburg RJ, Gelband H, Hoffman BF. Functional characteristics of the gating mechanism in the canine A-V conduction system. Circ Res 1971;28: 136–47.

39. Gouaux JL, Ashman R. Auricular fibrillation with aberration stimulating ventricular paroxysmal tachycardia. Am Heart J 1947;34:366–73.

40. Langendorf R, Pick A. Concealed intraventricular conduction in the human heart. Adv Cardiol 1975; 14:40–50.

41. Denker S, Shenasa M, Gilbert C, et al. Effects of abrupt changes in cycle length on refractoriness of the His-Purkinje system in man. Circulation 1983; 67:60–8.

42. Akhtar M, Denker S, Lehmann M, et al. Effects of sudden cycle length alteration on refractoriness of human His-Purkinje system and ventricular myocardium. In: Zipes D, Jalife J, editors. Cardiac electrophysiology and arrhythmias. New York: Grune & Stratton Publishers; 1985. p. 399.

43. Akhtar M, Damato AN, Batsford WP, et al. Unmasking and conversion of gap phenomenon in the human heart. Circulation 1974;49:624–30.

44. Akhtar M, Damato AN, Caracta AR, et al. The gap phenomena during retrograde conduction in man. Circulation 1974;49:811–7.

45. Damato AN, Akhtar M, Ruskin J, et al. Gap phenomena: anterograde and retrograde. In: Wellens HJJ, Lie KI, Janse MJ, editors. The conduction system of the heart. Philadelphia: Lea & Febiger (Springer); 1976. p. 504–28.

46. Lehmann MH, Denker S, Mahmud R, et al. Functional His-Purkinje system behavior during sudden ventricular rate acceleration in man. Circulation 1983;68:767–75.

47. Akhtar M, Damato AN, Ruskin JN, et al. Characteristics and coexistence of two forms of ventricular echo phenomena. Am Heart J 1976;92:174–82.

48. Greene HL, Reid PR, Schaeffer AH. The repetitive ventricular response in man. A predictor of sudden death. N Engl J Med 1978;299:729–34.

49. Ruskin JN, DiMarco JP, Garan H. Repetitive responses to single ventricular extrastimuli in patients with serious ventricular arrhythmias: incidence and clinical significance. Circulation 1981;63:767–72.

50. Mason JW. Repetitive beating after single ventricular extrastimuli: incidence and prognostic significance in patients with recurrent ventricular tachycardia. Am J Cardiol 1980;45:1126–31.

51. Akhtar M. Editorial: the clinical significance of the repetitive ventricular response. Circulation 1981;63: 773–5.

52. Farshidi A, Michelson EL, Greenspan AM, et al. Repetitive responses to ventricular extrastimuli: incidence, mechanism and significance. Am Heart J 1980;100:59–68.

53. Avitall B, McKinnie J, Jazayeri M, et al. Induction of ventricular fibrillation versus monomorphic ventricular tachycardia during programmed stimulation: role of premature beat conduction delay. Circulation 1992;85:1271–8.

54. Akhtar M. Supraventricular tachycardias: electrophysiologic mechanisms, diagnosis and pharmacologic therapy. In: Josephson ME, Wellens HJJ, editors. Tachycardias: mechanisms, diagnosis and treatment. Philadelphia: Lea and Febiger (Springer); 1984. p. 137.

55. Mahmud R, Denker S, Lehmann MH, et al. The effect of AV sequential pacing in patients with no ventriculoatrial conduction. J Am Coll Cardiol 1984;4: 273–7.

Part II

Part II

Human His-Purkinje System
Abnormalities of Conduction, Rhythm Disorders and Case Studies

Masood Akhtar, MD, FACC, FACP, MACP, FAHA, FHRS

KEYWORDS

- His-Purkinje system • Electrophysiology • Pathology • AV blocks • Fascicular tachycardias
- Bundle branch reentry • Supraventricular tachycardias • Preexcitation syndromes

KEY POINTS

- With many arrhythmias, an abnormal His-Purkinje system (HPS) is either the primary culprit or is intimately involved.
- Among the nontachycardia situations, bundle branch block and its various manifestations are discussed.
- A higher degree of block such as 2:1, 3:1 and intermittent second-degree block and some issues regarding their definition are also discussed.
- Junctional premature complexes, automatic junctional tachycardia, idiopathic left posterior inferior fascicular tachycardia, multiform left post inferior fascicular tachycardia are presented, and bundle branch reentry tachycardia (BBR).
- The role of the HPS in the setting of supraventricular tachycardia and AP is also addressed.

ABNORMALITIES OF THE HIS-PURKINJE SYSTEM

Covered under this title are all underlying pathologic/organic (structural) myocardial and valvular diseases with His-Purkinje involvement and causing patient symptoms. Also included are electrocardiographic (ECG) abnormalities or symptoms related to the His-Purkinje system (HPS), even if there is no cardiac structural pathology per se. An example of this is seen in patients with supraventricular tachycardia (SVT), where the HPS is not directly responsible but participates in the arrhythmia. The pediatric population is not discussed here, particularly if there is a congenital structural heart disease.

BUNDLE BRANCH BLOCK

One of the most benign HPS abnormalities is bundle branch block (BBB), fascicular block without any associated pathologies and no related symptoms.[1–3] Similarly, having incomplete BBB is not considered normal and hence may be mentioned in this context.

1. Right BBB (RBBB) or left BBB (LBBB) on the baseline ECG is abnormal. For most adults with RBBB with no cardiac or pulmonary pathology, there is no change in the prognosis, but the various ECG forms where RBBB presents itself need some clarification. Rate-related BBB is typically defined as the development of RBBB or LBBB at a certain rate acceleration achieved by pacing or exercise, or a critical rate slowing (**Figs. 1** and **2**), and so on.[2–5] The tachycardia-related or so-called phase 3 block means that the relative refractory period (RRP) or effective refractory period (ERP) of the bundle branch (BB) reaches at a certain rate, and normalizes at a slower rate.

Aurora Cardiovascular Services, Aurora Sinai/Aurora St. Luke's Medical Centers, University of Wisconsin School of Medicine and Public Health, 2801 W. Kinnickinnic River Parkway, Suite 777, Milwaukee, WI, USA
E-mail address: publishing@aurora.org

Card Electrophysiol Clin 8 (2016) 683–742
http://dx.doi.org/10.1016/j.ccep.2016.07.004
1877-9182/16/© 2016 Elsevier Inc. All rights reserved.

The rate does not have to qualify as a tachycardia (see **Fig. 1**).[3] The implication is that an involved or affected BB has a prolonged refractory period and does not shorten at shorter cycle length (CL) as occurs normally. This may happen because of some underlying cardiac, valvular, myocardial, or pulmonary pathology, or because of the diseased HPS itself. The reason rate-related BBB is considered abnormal is that, when a particular rate is reached, BBB will occur and at that rate, or at a faster rate, the impulse is unlikely to conduct normally. It could happen with atrial tachycardia, exercise, or pacing, but the underlying process causing it may not be very obvious. With physiologic or functional BBB, in contrast, the BB or fascicle can conduct normally at the same or faster rate at which it conducts aberrantly. Compared with RBBB without associated pathology, LBBB carries a less favorable prognosis and this is somewhat of a change from the past.[6–10]

For the most part, RBBB appearing during exercise produces no symptoms, but some patients who develop LBBB during exercise lose the ability to continue the exercise at the same intensity and may even have chest pain and feel exhausted. For years there was a perception that LBBB without structural heart disease[a] was benign. This is no longer the case. Although it may not apply to everyone, it is clearer than previously appreciated:

That the start of LBBB during activity (exercise, etc) may be reflective of underlying cardiac disease and may create an appreciable loss of energy in some patients.[11,12] These patients could progress to a stage where they have LBBB with every complex. At that point, they may not feel the abrupt change during exercise. Some could, however, gradually deteriorate to a state of left ventricular (LV) dysfunction (owing to myocardial dysynchrony), requiring intervention.[8–10]

Without intervention, patients may deliberately reduce the level of exercise when the LBBB occurs. Sometimes, the caregiver has to slow their heart rate with pharmaceutical agents to avoid the rate at which they develop symptoms. In the past, mainly patients with newly discovered LBBB were considered as harboring underlying coronary artery disease. At present, all one can say is that the LBBB is a predictor of higher mortality, particularly when associated with left axis deviation. Constant right ventricular (RV) pacing and/or spontaneous LBBB may lead to LV dysfunction in some cases, which may need biventricular pacing.[8–15] Although it is not clear at the moment what the preferred pacing mode should be, biventricular pacing may turn out to be a logical choice for many patients needing permanent pacemakers in the future.

At the other end of the spectrum there is the so-called phase 4 or bradycardia-dependent BBB. Here, a longer than prevailing CL may be needed to expose the BBB pattern. It is not clear what exact length of long CL is needed to reveal the underlying abnormality (see **Figs. 1** and **2**). Some of the examples shown were excessively long CL (see **Fig. 2**).[5] The proposed mechanism is that a propagating impulse encounters lower resting membrane potential (hypopolarization) owing to spontaneous phase 4 depolarization caused by a long pause, hence the term. In a traumatic BBB, it simply takes a longer than normal CL to see phase 4. For example, the first complex after a Wenckebach block in the atrioventricular (AV) node may be sufficient to reveal bradycardia-dependent BBB (**Fig. 3**).[16] Looking at both phase 3 and phase 4 block in the HPS, it seems to be an almost universal phenomenon in chronic situations at the early stages of BBB; however, at times, extreme rates may be necessary.[5]

2. Permanent/persistent BBB. It raises a natural question whether all BBB or HPS blocks go through phase 3 and 4 stages before becoming permanent/persistent BBB: it is difficult to distinguish between the 2 terms because permanency gives the impression that the BBB is always present. Because patients are not monitored at all times, "persistence" is a preferable term. For RBBB, there may be minimal underlying pathology such as patchy fibrosis, local calcium deposition, or more extensive, that is, RV, hypertrophy, dilated cardiomyopathy, pulmonary hypertension, or pulmonary valve disease to explain it. There also is not a serious long-term sequelae associated with isolated RBBB other than perhaps some diagnostic confusion. When the first ECG in an individual shows RBBB, it is often referred to as preexisting, and in otherwise symptomatic patients it may initiate some clinical workup. The presence of a persistent LBBB should always be taken as if it is associated with some LV pathology,

---

[a]The term structural heart disease has been used by electrophysiologists for more than 30 years to describe any anatomically identifiable heart disease including coronary heart disease and cardiomyopathies, and so on, which is somewhat different as compared with its use in the general cardiology community.

which is likely in the majority of cases. At the very least, essential hypertension, LV outflow pathologies such as aortic valve stenosis, hypertrophic cardiomyopathy (obstructive or nonobstructive), dilated idiopathic cardiomyopathy, coronary artery disease, or HPS disease per se. The exact role of increased intracavitary pressures, myocardial stretch, and so on, if any, have not been demonstrated clearly as contributing to either of the persistent BBB. Isolated fascicular block is likely to be a result of some HPS abnormality, but an underlying myocardial process cannot be excluded completely. Patients with isolated LBBB need LV function evaluation and exclusion of conditions likely to be associated with LBBB before it can be labeled as a lone (or isolated) LBBB. Furthermore, even asymptomatic patients should have at least 1 follow-up cardiac ultrasound examination in 6 to 12 months for evidence of any LV functional deterioration.

3. Another intriguing observation under the pathology umbrella is the so-called fatigue phenomenon in the HPS.[17,18] Assuming no abrupt CL changes are involved, the term fatigue seems appropriate (for lack of a better term) in the following situation. With a normal baseline conduction, at constant atrial pacing at moderate rates, for example 400 to 800 ms CL, LBBB or RBBB may develop after several complexes show normal conduction and without a change in CL. Furthermore, in the setting of a nonspecific intraventricular conduction delay (IVCD) at baseline, constant CL V pacing or spontaneous (ventricular tachycardia) VT, a BBB appears at the termination of pacing and may last for several CL. These 2 responses will not occur with functional, rate-related, or persistent BBB, making it a unique entity, the cause for which remains unclear.

4. Complete and incomplete BBB are commonly used terms to describe QRS duration of 120 ms or greater (with complete) in association with a BBB. The fact of the matter is that no width of QRS can determine the completeness of a BBB. That is, AV conduction along the BB is almost always present unless one damages a bundle with a catheter or other form of ablation, or some serious trauma. Because many times it is simply a conduction delay rather than block, the term BBB pattern is a more appropriate one. A 40-ms asynchrony of conduction between the 2 bundles (40–50 ms is the transseptal conduction time) will be more than sufficient to produce a complete BBB pattern.

5. Unless coexisting with a BBB, isolated fascicular block does not prolong the QRS a great deal because the Purkinje network of the various divisions of the LBB has extensive connections. Furthermore, the 2 ventricles are still being activated simultaneously and transseptal conduction is not involved.

6. One of the criteria used to interpret LBBB versus nonspecific IVCD defect is based on the absence of a Q wave in lead I, AVL, and, to a lesser extent, V_6. Anatomic studies have indicated that the septal division of LBB can be a separate and sometimes the largest division. Its contribution as an independent fascicle is rarely recognized. At this juncture, it is tempting to postulate that the so-called incomplete LBBB, which essentially means a loss of Q wave in lead I with minimal QRS widening may simply be a pure form of septal divisional block and conversely the presence of Q wave in lead I should not exclude the diagnosis of complete LBBB if the QRS width is greater than 120 ms. Interestingly, many patients with nonspecific IVCD of the LBB type have long HV intervals, suggesting HPS disease. This will again be discussed in the section on bundle branch reentrant (BBR) tachycardia.

7. Bidirectional block. In the BBs, somewhat akin to complete versus incomplete anterograde block, the retrograde counterpart may precede, follow, or coexist with anterograde BBB and/or fascicular block. The latter could play a role in providing sufficient delay (not block) to create suitable environments conducive to the occurrence of interfascicular or BBR VT. Bidirectional BBB or simply the retrograde component is not difficult to prove if looked for. Isolated examples of retrograde BBB are often observed with spontaneous ventricular premature complex or during RV pacing induced LBBB (**Figs. 4** and **5**). This finding is one explanation for differences in VA intervals when the switch occurs from ipsilateral to contralateral origin of premature complexes. This change is localized to the HPS (VH) rather than the AV node (ie, HA). Similarly, ventricular extrastimulation ipsilateral and contralateral to the BBB, respectively, may reveal normal intraventricular conduction or retrograde BBB or delay depending on the chamber paced and concomitant anterograde BBB (**Figs. 6** and **7**).[16] Although the observations mentioned are of interest, their role in clinical situations is limited, but the important role of unidirectional or bidirectional BBB in SVT and VT will become clear later.

8. The site of block in BBB. The exact incident of block site with pathologic BBB is not known in all the patients, but the following observations have been made. El-Sherif and colleagues[19] in an experimental model and Narula[20] in humans showed that a lesion in the His bundle (HB) produced classic changes of a BBB downstream. These investigators explained this finding on the basis of longitudinal dissociation in the HB. In essence, it meant that certain fibers within the HB are predestined to continue as BBs or fascicles. Pacing proximal to the lesion produced QRS morphology and axis exactly as the baseline sinus rhythm, whereas a few millimeters distally, pacing completely normalized the QRS and the left axis (**Figs. 8** and **9**).[20] In the current way of thinking, a better explanation for these fascinating findings is more likely to be anisotropic conduction (**Fig. 10**),[21,22] which will provide sufficient delay to produce a BBB because the HPS impulse feed distal to the lesion may be delayed sufficiently and can be overcome by pacing distally. A dramatic example of spontaneous proximal RBBB (with RB recording) and complete interruption of conduction is displayed in a patient with preexisting RBBB (**Fig. 11**).[23] A block is between H and RB such that the sinus impulse reaches the LV via LBB (LB-V of 25 ms) and retrograde activates RB (distal RB precedes proximal) with long LV distal (see **Fig. 11**). This is an example of the magnitude of spontaneous conduction delay that can exist in the proximal HPS over a relatively short distance.

9. Trifascicular nature of LBB. Ever since Mauricio Rosenbaum and his colleagues described their brilliant findings, there has been an assumption that left bundle has 2 fascicles. Many investigators subsequently have presented evidence of various degrees to suggest that there are more than 2 divisions and therefore the terms fascicular and/or divisional block has been preferred over the term hemiblock.[23,24] However, trifascicular LBB should not be confused with trifascicular AV block. The latter term evolved when there was a combination of 2 fascicles showing conduction delay and/or block and additional PR interval prolongation. This was thought to reflect the conduction delay in the third fascicle (ie, 3 out of 3, not 3 out of 4 [LBB being trifascicular]). This line of thinking did not pan out because, in many cases, the PR prolongation was owing to AV nodal delay and not additional HPS conduction delay and/or block.

Some of the aspects of LBB fascicles need further discussion.

a. A component of vertical orientation has been used in the definition of fascicular block because the diagnosis of divisional block was primarily made by the QRS orientation in bipolar limb leads. So the anterior division became anterior–superior, and the posterior has been termed posterior–inferior. The anterior and posterior QRS orientation has not been incorporated in the diagnosis of divisional block to the present day and is not used clinically. So why use an anatomic term when no criteria have been developed for clinical diagnosis in horizontal leads? A superior and inferior axis terminology will suffice.

b. The presence of a septal division of the left bundle as a separate division has been implied by several investigators[25]; however, an active clinical role has not been convincingly demonstrated, except recently.[24,26] Although pathologic specimens clearly show the division, its clinical electrophysiologic manifestation has been marginalized. There are several pieces of evidence that indicate an active role. The diagnosis of incomplete LBB, for example, has not been clarified. Although it cannot be proven, it would not be out of context to state again that the loss of Q wave in lead I actually represents a pure septal divisional conduction delay or block and it should be expressed as such rather than a vague term such as incomplete LBBB, which actually takes away the focus from septal division and projects it onto the entire LBB system.

c. The recent description of fascicular tachycardias by Sung and colleagues[24] strongly supports the trifascicular nature of LBB, even though recording from the septal division was not provided, and in the diagram, the septal pattern was shown to participate only in a retrograde direction.[24]

d. Almost by chance, we ran into some evidence that brought together the trifascicular nature of the left BB and active participation of septal division in LV activation more convincingly than before.[26] When the right BB (RBB) was accidentally traumatized or ablated (during ablation of concealed anteroseptal AP), the postablation 12-lead ECG showed a complete RBBB pattern and no other changes compared with the baseline, which was a normal 12-lead ECG (**Fig. 12**).[26] However, when a RBB ablation was done in patients with sustained BB reentry (abnormal HPS with prolonged HV at the baseline) many new, different, and unexpected findings were noted on 12-lead ECG. Twelve of 14 patients developed a new pathologic Q wave in lead

V_1 and sometimes in lead V_2 (9 of 14; **Figs. 13** and **14**). Four of 14 patients developed a left superior shift of the axis, which was greater than 45° different from baseline (see **Fig. 13**). Another 3 of 14 patients developed inferior axis shift of greater than 45° (see **Fig. 14**.) These patients who already had a long HV interval had further prolongation (mean, 30 ms), suggesting that RBB was still contributing to ventricular activation before ablation, even if they had complete RBBB pattern at the baseline with prolonged HV interval. Because most patients had IVCD of the LBBB type, that is, Q wave in lead I and V_6 plus an LBBB pattern before RB ablation, an increase in HV after ablation of the RBB implied that some part of the LBB and its fascicles were retrogradely penetrated via the RBB.

These changes after ablation in patients with BBR (where no part of the LBB was touched) can be best explained as follows. After RBB ablation, it is assumed that RBB did not contribute any longer to ventricular activation. Therefore, the LV activation exclusively occurred via the LBB with asynchronous delay along its divisions, as would be expected. This also unmasked functioning trifascicular LBB system as to why so many changes occurred on the left side after ablation of the RBB only. The LBB conduction delay in its 3 divisions was not equal, so that the pathologic septal new Q wave development was owing to greater conduction delay in the septal division in some patients relative to the other patients who did not show this QRS morphologic change. In a similar way, the right or left axis deviation noticed in a high percentage of patients suggested greater conduction delay in the respective fascicles compared with the remaining one or two. It is not logical to assume that the 3 divisions of the left bundle would have equal conduction delay. If that was the case, other than prolongation of the HV interval and development of the RBBB, no other changes would be noticed on the postablation 12-lead ECG, which did happen in 2 of the 14 patients. To explain these findings, it is hypothesized that before ablation, the native supraventricular impulse entered the left ventricle retrograde via the RBB, and partially penetrated the divisions of the LBB. This would have resulted in masking the full contribution of ventricular activation via the LBB if any. This is an important electrophysiologic concept and will be discussed again to explain some clinical tachycardias. This is further supported by the fact that the preablation ECG, in most cases, showed a nonspecific IVCD of the LBBB type. The baseline HV prolongation that all of these patients (with BBR)

display attests to the diseased nature of the HPS in this clinical situation. Another rather important observation reinforces the presence of a septal division and serious doubts regarding the true nature of nonspecific IVCD. Is it intramyocardial or HPS conduction delay or both? Further HV prolongation with RBB ablation suggests a contribution by the HPS to an IVCD complex, which may be simply LBBB with lesser delay in the septal division.

ATRIOVENTRICULAR BLOCK AND THE HIS-PURKINJE SYSTEM

Traditionally, the AV conduction, when abnormal, is classified into 3 categories, that is, first, second, and third degrees. To put it in another way: (1) prolonged AV conduction, (2) intermittent AV conduction, and (3) no AV conduction, respectively. From an electrophysiologic standpoint, second-degree AV block or intermittent AV conduction and blocks are physiologically and academically the most challenging and interesting, and more detailed at the outset. Traditionally, the second-degree AV block is subdivided it into 3 types, that is, Mobitz types I and II (**Figs. 15** and **16**), and a higher or more advanced degree of block.[27,28] During the higher degree there may be 2:1 3:1, or 4:1 AV conduction ratio or multiple P waves followed by a spontaneous or paced QRS (**Figs. 17** and **18**).[29] Depending on the number of blocked P waves before a QRS, it is easy to confuse this with transient third-degree AV block (see **Figs. 16–18**). I do not know the generally accepted definition of so-called transient/paroxysmal/intermittent AV block with multiple P waves block—is it second or third degree? To my way of thinking, when a number of P waves block in the HPS, but the episodes end with a conducted QRS it is second-degree versus idioventricular escape mechanism; it is third degree unless one reserves the definition of complete AV block as a permanent form of block only.

Mobitz I AV block is also referred to as AV Wenckebach phenomenon (WP), is the progressive prolongation of the PR interval ending with a block of a P wave and then the cycle is repeated (see **Fig. 15**).[30] The second conducted P wave has the longest increment of PR within the cycle, such that during the blocked P wave the R-R is the longest and subsequently there is R–R shortening until the next block of the P wave. The latter part of the definition is useful when the origin of impulse is not visible, such as in sinoatrial WP. Distinction between Mobitz I versus II AV block is often equated with site of block, that is, AV nodal versus HPS, respectively (see **Fig. 16**). In this regard there are multiple issues with the completeness of Mobitz I or WP definition that have been talked about but never formalized. These are that (1) There is no mention of the absolute length of the PR interval, (2) no importance is given to the duration of preblock and postblock PR interval, and (3) if the PR is very prolonged, such as ≥ 350 ms, would a sudden block of P wave be considered a Mobitz II (**Fig. 16B**) (4) On the other hand, Mobitz type II is often Mobitz type I in the HPS (see **Fig. 15B, C**). The reason it is not interpreted as such is because the change in the HPS delay from beat to beat is often very subtle and not measurable on the surface ECG (see **Fig. 15C**). What was said for infrahisian blocks applies to intrahisian blocks as well where the baseline PR and QRS are often normal but could be aberrant (see **Fig. 15**). Based on current understanding and ongoing discussion, it is reasonable to conclude that (1) the AV is relatively benign when located in the AV node, (2) the so-called Mobitz II is often WP phenomenon (see **Fig. 15C**) in the HPS when there is subtle PR to PR change but obvious in some patients (**Fig. 15B**), and (3) both Mobitz II or I in the HPS require a pacemaker sooner or later, but that cannot be stated for the AV node. Some improvements to distinguish HPS versus AV nodal blocks on surface ECG are suggested. These could be helpful and sometimes may be even more helpful than usual criteria for the diagnosis. (1) If the absolute length of PR is greater than 350 ms, it is likely to be a block in the AV node regardless of the degree. (2) A subtle Mobitz I block is usually in the HPS. This possibility increases if the conducted PR is normal and QRS shows BBB or bifascicular block. (3) When the block occurs during Mobitz I and the PR change from before the block to after the block is more than 100 ms, it points toward the AV node. (4) The intermittent AV block, particularly when several P waves are blocked in a row, could be in the AV node (usually vagal) or in the HPS. The latter is perhaps a more serious situation than second- or third-degree HPS block. Ironic as it may sound, some of these patients with intermittent AV block maintain a 1:1 P QRS relationship for years.[31] Therefore, an ECG done years after pacemaker implant may still show 1:1 conduction and the physicians wonder if the pacemaker was necessary (see **Figs. 17** and **18**). Considering the seriousness of the block when it does occur, this is the very population where a permanent pacemaker is absolutely necessary. With 1:1 conduction for a long period of time in these patients with intermittent second- or third-degree AV block, some have been led to believe that in this particular population the pacemaker is overused (see **Figs. 17–19; Fig. 20**).[32] This is a clinically risky way of thinking with serious consequences when the block occurs, the timing of which is unpredictable (see **Figs. 17–20**). In this patient population, when symptomatic pacemaker implantation is a straightforward decision. Documentation of block site in patients with intermittent symptomatic AV block will require some documentation, but may not be necessary. A rather simple method is to expose HPS block is exercise. If a patient develops AV block during exercise or even drops a single QRS when the P wave is on time, the site of block is likely to be in the HPS. But if a doubt still exists, intracardiac recordings may be necessary along with some provocation such as atrial pacing and/or intravenous procainamide (up to10 mg/kg) to demonstrate AV block in the HPS (**Figs. 21** and **22**).[16] Some of these patients have bidirectional block in the HPS (see **Fig. 20**).

First-degree AV block, in general, is not taken very seriously, even if there is concomitant aberrant conduction, as long as the patient is asymptomatic. Patients who are symptomatic such as those with syncope or presyncope should be further evaluated and HPS block occurring intermittently should be excluded. However, PR prolongation per se may cause a symptomatic condition regardless of the location of the conduction delay, that is, the AV node versus HPS. Here, the key reason will be the actual length of the PR interval. For example, a patient with a PR interval of greater than 350 ms may have very limited capacity to exercise, because the P may encroach upon the previous T wave, unless the PR shortens in the process of exercise. Some of this has become more apparent since radiofrequency catheter ablation/modification of the AV node was initiated. Before that, if a patient was symptomatic and had a long PR interval, the effects of any agents such as propranolol, calcium channel blockers, and so on, had to be excluded. Aside from these considerations, presently the PR may prolong inadvertently during ablation of slow AV nodal pathway or deliberate ablation of the fast pathway done earlier in the experience. PR prolongation that occurs this way is unlikely to significantly shorten with exercise. Thus, the patient's palpitations are now replaced by fatigue.[33] Energy level drops, exercise capacity is reduced, and the patient is as unhappy as they were before—for different reasons, of course. This is why this possibility must be explained to the patient before the procedure, because it is always possible, even though rare currently, because of experience in slow pathway ablation. If PR prolongation is owing to HPS conduction delay and the patient has serious symptoms such as syncope and nothing else is found to explain them, a pacemaker is indicated.[34] However, other conditions, particularly VT, should be diligently sought, because they often turn out to be the cause of unexplained syncope.[34,35] As it stands now, someone with presyncope or syncope, a low left ventricular ejection fraction (LVEF; ≤35) and no obvious cause, an implantable cardioverter defibrillator is the appropriate treatment which also provides backup bradycardia pacing.[36]

Third-Degree Atrioventricular Block (No Atrioventricular Conduction)

The underlying causes of third-degree heart block are many, including coronary artery disease, cardiomyopathy, Chagas' disease, and Lenegre's disease. These may cause HPS blocks both proximally and distally. However, some conditions tend to produce AV block proximally. These include valvular pathology either de novo or with prosthetic valve or valvular calcification. The diseases that were just mentioned are by no means a complete list.

The third-degree block in the HPS, when it occurs initially, a series of P waves may block (see **Fig. 19**) before the escape rhythm emerges, because these subsidiary pacemakers have been dormant throughout life. Therefore, the initial pause could be quite long and produce symptoms of presyncope, syncope, or occasionally long QT interval, which could cause torsade des pointes. It may be of interest to know that initial description of torsade des pointes was made in the setting of AV block.[37] When third-degree block is established, the subsidiary pacemakers could be quite stable and continue to function for years, albeit the rates will be slow. Both ventricles are capable of sustaining a stable ventricular rhythm from these subsidiary pacemakers. Once these pacemakers are suppressed with other means such as artificial pacing or nonsustained VT, it may be difficult to wean off pacing owing to overdrive suppression and sometimes may take several minutes to do so. These situations have only arisen in patients who deny symptoms with third-degree heart block and can function. The denial may be either owing to socioeconomic reasons, the availability of a competent facility within a manageable distance. Some patients feel that the reduced energy level is related to aging or fear of the pacemaker owing to various reasons, including having heard horror stories about the outcome in patients with pacemakers. Once they get the permanent pacemaker, their energy level improves and then the patient asks, why did you not do this earlier?

Having recommended a permanent pacemaker implant, the second question asked presently is whether RV apical pacing is a wise choice, because some patients develop deterioration of LV function.[14,15] It seems that more and more patients are having conversion to biventricular pacing from single site pacing in the right ventricle and this trend may continue.

The 2 locations of third-degree AV block are the AV node and the HPS, and only the HPS will be discussed herein. No one has recorded multiple electrodes placed along the HPS to confirm either the site of block or the origin of subsidiary pacemakers. There is a perception that, because the rate of the pacemaker is slow (ie, 20–40 ms), it is located distally in the HPS. Regardless, such slow rates are a sufficient reason to implant a permanent pacemaker. Invariably the experience of the operators is that the patient feels better with bradycardia support.

PSEUDO ATRIOVENTRICULAR BLOCK AND THE HIS-PURKINJE SYSTEM
His Bundle Premature Complexes

Although the HB premature complexes can simulate first-, second-, and third-degree AV block and various other phenomenon (**Fig. 23**), depending on the timing of these premature complexes, the most commonly published examples mimic Mobitz type II (**Fig. 24**).[37,38] If discharge of the HB bundle premature discharge is close to the previous QRS, it is unable to activate the ventricle in the forward direction (see **Fig. 24**A). At the same time, retrograde block in the AV node makes the oncoming sinus p wave block unexpectedly (simulates Mobitz type II).[37] The patient may not have extensive disease of any other organ or even cardiac tissue. The HB, however, could be affected by ventricular disease, prosthetic valve or HPS abnormality. The pseudo AV block can be suspected from surface ECG by the observation that these premature complexes may activate the ventricle intermittently with narrow or aberrant QRS. If the premature HB discharge reaches the atria it will produce an inverted P wave, which is also narrow (see **Fig. 23**). The reason for the latter is that the retrograde impulse activates the atria in a divergent fashion as it exits from the AV node. Both atria are simultaneously depolarized in almost one-half the duration of the normal P wave. If QRS occurs at the same time, this analysis of P wave will be difficult because the P may be obscured by the QRS or distorted within the ST-T segment (see **Fig. 24**C). The ultimate proof of its presence can be established with HB recordings.

Isoarrhythmic Atrioventricular Dissociation

In this situation, the atria and ventricle are depolarized by separate and independent foci. The PR interval can vary, but is fixed for a certain period of time, although it is shorter than the PR when it is conducted (**Fig. 25**). The ventricle has its own rhythm, but marching along at the same rate. There is no block in either AV or VA direction, P wave can conduct to the QRS and the ventricular impulse can reach the atria, given the time. This results in 1 form of AV dissociation with 2 independent foci. This might be a good moment to point out that the expression "AV dissociation" is like saying the patient has congestive heart failure to a cardiologist, because neither one of these address the causes. The 4 types of AV dissociation are (1) AV block, (2) VA block (as occurs in VT or V pacing), (3) isoarrhythmic AV dissociation where there is no AV or VA block, and (4) the slowing of primary rhythm and emergence of subsidiary pacemaker rhythm and linking mostly by interference above the site of subsidiary pacemaker to sustain.[39]

TACHYCARDIAS AND THE HIS-PURKINJE SYSTEM

It seems logical to start with the tachycardias originating in the HPS (ie, ventricular) then move on to SVT with secondary involvement of HPS.

Tachycardias Originating Within the His-Purkinje System

1. Automatic junctional tachycardia. This tachycardia most likely arises from the HB and the underlying mechanism is not reentry because it cannot be initiated or terminated with programmed stimulation. The latter is characteristic of all reentrant tachycardias.[40,41] Abnormal automaticity has been suggested as the underlying mechanism. The QRS complex is usually narrow, but can have aberrant conduction and somewhat irregular as the RR measurements go (**Fig. 26**). This is more common in younger individuals, but does occur in the older population. During the tachycardia there is AV dissociation, which is helpful in its diagnosis. The closest differential is 1:2 response in patients with dual AV nodal physiology (**Fig. 27**).[41–44] On the HB electrogram, the H-V interval is normal or may be prolonged and the exact frequency of its occurrence is uncertain. It may respond to pharmaceutical agents that have a suppressing effect on the HPS. At this point, a symptomatic and recurrent automatic junctional tachycardia is best treated with ablation of the focus and it can be done without creating AV block and, if the AV block occurs, permanent pacemaker will be required. Other tachycardias mimicking the automatic variety include AV nodal reentry and accelerated AV junctional rhythm, which may exceed 100 beats/min (**Fig. 28**). The latter is generally seen in clinical scenarios with higher adrenergic drive, usually no therapy is needed and as the patient recovers the tachycardia subsides. If it produces hemodynamic instability, the rate can be slowed down by class I agents and, if necessary, class III agents such as amiodarone. Although beta-blockers will effectively counter the adrenergic drive, they may not be advisable in all patients. The other differential is the common AV nodal reentry, which is characterized by meeting all the reentry criteria. There is a 1:1 PQRS relationship, and the onset of retrograde P wave is simultaneous with the QRS such that the P wave is rarely identifiable on surface ECG. Occasionally, there is a 2:1 H-A block (retrograde) but never AV dissociation.[45] How much a part of the atrium is necessary to sustain this tachycardia has been a controversial subject, but it is conceivable that a small rim of atrium around the AV node may participate in the circuit even with apparent HA block. The published examples of so-called AV nodal reentry with AV dissociation are more compatible with automatic junctional tachycardia, 1:2 AV response, BB reentry or fascicular reentry rather than AV nodal reentry, so the distinction is relatively easy if there is AV dissociation during the junctional tachycardia.[44–46] Another tachycardia that would be almost impossible to distinguish would be intra-HB reentry, a convincing example of which I have not seen or demonstrated so far, although it will at least follow reentry criteria. Finally, a narrow QRS tachycardia arising from the septal division retrogradely enters both left anterior superior and posterior inferior fascicles anterogradely, an example of which will be shown under multiform fascicular tachycardias. Although symptoms of palpitations and near syncope are common, sudden arrhythmic death is rare in the adult population

2. Left posterior fascicular tachycardia.[47–50] This particular arrhythmia is also known as idiopathic left VT, sometimes referred to as verapamil sensitive. The typical 12-lead ECG shows a RBBB and left axis deviation pattern (see **Fig. 28**). The onset of the QRS is somewhat rapid and the total QRS duration tends to be narrower than a myocardial VT. Although there

was some controversy regarding the mechanism as to whether it is triggered activity, mostly because of responsiveness to verapamil and atrial inducibility or reentry, but more recently it has been established as reentry (**Fig. 29**). The criteria of reentry that is initiation and termination with programmed electrical stimulation are not. Definition of the circuit with entrainment from the site of origin posterior inferior part of the left ventricle has left little doubt about the mechanism and the reentry circuit demonstration recently is quite convincing. There is usually no underlying structural heart disease. The LV function is normal, and symptoms of palpitations, syncope, and presyncope are not uncommon; however, sudden arrhythmic death is rare. The tachycardia does respond to intravenous verapamil and somewhat more inconsistently to oral calcium channel blockers. At this time, the best and preferred treatment is ablation of part of the circuit and this can be done without affecting the conduction in the posterior/inferior fascicle. The Purkinje potential precedes the QRS by variable interval and is the usual site of ablation (**Fig. 30**).

3. Multiform fascicular tachycardia.[24] Recently, Sung and colleagues[24] described 6 cases out of 823 patients with VT that fit the criteria of multiform fascicular tachycardia an incidence of less than 1%. Four of 6 patients had no structural heart disease and in all cases the HB preceded the QRS and the tachycardias could be entrained. The tachycardias have various morphologies, suggesting 3 divisions of the LB actively participating and the RB either passively or actively engaged.[24] Three of the 6 also had narrow QRS tachycardia, suggesting the presence of retrograde conduction via a septal division. No recordings from the fascicles were made and the analysis is based on the HB timing, QRS morphology, and entrainment. The existence of retrograde septal fascicular conduction was necessary in all morphologies shown in **Fig. 31**. The treatment was mostly catheter ablation and the most successful sites were the respective fascicles, but resulted in BBR unless the septal fascicle was ablated. One patient was treated with pharmacologic agents. The finding reproduced by the authors strengthens the evidence of active participation of a septal division of LBB in these clinical tachycardias.

4. BBR tachycardia.[51–61] This topic was partly covered earlier to describe the physiologic phenomenon of BBR usually lasting for 1 complex with spontaneous termination in normal

individuals.[52] The spontaneous termination is primarily because these are patients with normal HPS conduction, quick accommodation, and, hence, self-limiting. The realization that to sustain this phenomenon you need an abnormal HPS that, when present, may lead to a sustained tachycardia initially called reentry HPS now mostly referred to as BBR.[57–61] The typical patient has dilated cardiomyopathy (ischemic or nonischemic),[53–55] nonspecific IVCD, and prolonged HPS conduction (HV interval). The baseline rhythm is sinus or atrial fibrillation. The QRS shows a LBBB type of IVCD on the surface ECG but occasionally an incomplete to complete RBBB pattern (**Figs. 32–35**). Nonetheless, as has been pointed out previously, the so-called complete BBB patterns do not reflect a block but more frequently conduction delay, an ideal milieu for BBR. These tachycardias are rapid and frequently cause syncope or convert into ventricular fibrillation and cardiac arrest. When the patient presents in sustained tachycardia, it shows a complete RBBB or LBBB pattern. Aside from the dilated cardiomyopathy, the tachycardia is also quite common with native valve disease or after valvular surgery or even if the LV function is completely normal.[55] The third disease often associated with BBR is myocardial dystrophy.[56] The tachycardia may also occur as a solo problem with simply HPS delay and no structural heart disease.[54,57,58] The circuit of reentry can be demonstrated clearly with concomitant recording of BB along with HB during sinus rhythm or any native supraventricular rhythm and during the spontaneous or induced tachycardias. The overall incidence of BBR among monomorphic tachycardia in our patient population is about 6%, but when there are other conditions present, such as idiopathic dilated cardiomyopathy, BBR in patients with inducible monomorphic VT increases to more than 25%. Similarly, in valvular disease, particularly after valve surgery, BBR frequency is also greater than 25% of inducible monomorphic VT. Because of the rapid rate of the BBR tachycardia, the VA conduction is seldom 1:1. A 2:1 or higher degree of block or AV dissociation is frequent. The HV interval is usually longer during BBR-VT than the sinus or any supraventricular rhythm, but at least theoretically can be shorter if the turnaround is lower than HB recording site.[55,56] BBR can be induced mostly with RV pacing, particularly with a short long sequence before the premature complex and occasionally with atrial pacing (**Figs. 36–38**). The following criteria have been observed in these patients repeatedly and used for the diagnosis.[52,61]

a. The HB potential precedes each QRS with HV interval equal to or longer than baseline rhythm and the initial QRS has rapid conduction owing to HPS activation.

b. During the first cycle, H_2V_3 is usually longer than baseline HV and reflects retrograde block in the HPS from V_2 (concealed conduction HPS).

c. When the HH and the following VV interval is measured, the HH change in cycle length always precedes the VV change (**Figs. 39** and **40**), indicating that the HB impulse is driving the ventricle and not the reverse.

d. If there is a block in the HPS, anterograde or retrograde, the VT terminates (see **Fig. 37**).

e. When the BB recordings have simultaneously recorded the subsequent QRS morphology is preceded by BB and HB sequence appropriate for that QRS configuration (see **Figs. 35–37**; **Fig. 41**).

f. Pacing-induced block in the HPS terminates the tachycardia, but if the HB is activated, it simply resets the BBR tachycardia (see **Fig. 38**).

g. The tachycardia can be entrained and the reentry criteria and the reentrant circuit can be demonstrated.

h. Ablation of right bundle or left BB will cure the VT (**Figs. 42–44**).[59,61]

Although the typical site of pacing during electrophysiologic studies is RV, the retrograde block of the RBB during premature stimulation occurs first and the impulse travels transseptally and reaches the HB retrograde via the LBB, which already has slow conduction (long HV baseline) and reenters the RB via the HB to start the tachycardia with an LBBB pattern. The axis could be normal, left, or right, depending on the retrograde conduction via 1 of the 3 fascicles. If the impulse activates the HB only via the anterior superior division, BBR-VT will have an LBBB and left axis morphology. Although it may be simpler that this type of reentry is cured with ablation of the RBB, the LBB in many cases has more conduction delay. For example, in a patient with a baseline IVCD of the LBBB type and a long HV interval, ablation of the LBB will be preferable. This will not change much of the underlying substrate and cure the tachycardia. However, traditionally RBB is relatively easy to ablate and has been done regardless of the QRS morphology. Several consequences of that are:

1. Further prolongation of the HV interval, confirming that RBBB was not complete despite meeting the ECG criteria. In patients with pre-existing RBBB and BBR, RBB ablation has minimum or no effect on the baseline HV and RBBB morphology.

2. There is development of new pathologic Q waves owing to septal divisional block. This is an important finding because it is the first time a pathologic role of septal division is demonstrated during life. A frequent shift in the axis owing to asynchronous conduction delay in the 3 fascicles of LBBB (see **Figs. 12–14**)[26] confirm the completion of RBBB owing to the ablative process that ventricular activation can only occur with LBB.

3. Complete AV block, which will then be treated with a permanent implantable pacemaker.

4. Interfascicular reentry of the same nature as BBR (ie, diseased HPS) involving the fascicles of LBB.[62] For reasons explained elsewhere in this paper, the occurrence of anterograde RBBB facilitates interfascicular reentry. This form of interfascicular reentry was not discussed under fascicular tachycardias because it occurs mostly in the setting of substrate for BBR. Complete interruption of RBB conduction by ablation or spontaneously with no impulse propagation via the RB to the ventricle (**Figs. 45–48**).[61] The underlying mechanism for this is that, when there is intact conduction via the RBB and the surface ECG shows either an LBBB pattern, nonspecific IVCD of the LBBB type, or incomplete RBBB, terminal parts of the 3 fascicles of the LBB are retrogradely penetrated, not allowing LV activation via the LB. Hence, there is no chance for interfascicular reentry in the absence of complete RBBB. This effect can also be altered by RV pacing, such that the paced impulse penetrates the fascicles of LBB from transseptal propagation and also prevent interfascicular reentry (see **Fig. 45**; **Fig. 46**). In the presence of complete RBBB, the LV fascicles are forced to conduct asynchronously, allowing manifestation of slow conduction and block one of the LB fascicles leading to sustained interfascicular reentry with right or left axis, depending on the circuit but concomitant RBBB, which is preexisting. In this context, the expression of complete RBBB is meant to denote complete interruption of RBB conduction and not just the surface ECG appearance. A fascicular ablation will cure this form of VT and still be able to produce a QRS via the other fascicles, albeit with prolongation of the PR interval (**Figs. 47** and **48**) owing to HPS conduction delay in the remaining unablated fascicles.

Supraventricular Tachycardia and the His-Purkinje System

It has been known for some time that, in patients with AP, when the ventricle free wall participates in reentrant circuits such as orthodromic or antidromic AV reentry, ipsilateral BBB (AP on the same side as the BBB) will prolong the VA interval.[62,63] Depending on the AV nodal characteristics, 1 of 2 scenarios can emerge. (1) If the AV node has no functional duality of pathways the cycle length of the tachycardia will prolong during BBB pattern, there is acceleration of rate during QRS normalization (**Fig. 46**).[62,63] The key factor here is the prolongation of VA interval with ipsilateral BBB. A change in the VA can also be detected with left anterior–superior fascicular block and pacing-induced BBB (V_3), of ventricular pacing per se.[64] Interestingly, superior axis further prolongs VA in comparison with LBBB plus normal or inferior axis (**Figs. 49–51**). (2) With coexistent dual AV nodal physiology, when the QRS normalizes after the BBB, the first VA interval will be shorter, which could engage the slow AV nodal pathway and in fact paradoxically prolong the CL of the narrow QRS tachycardia (**Fig. 52**).[46] Up to 15% of patients with functioning AP also have sustained AV nodal reentry of the common variety. In the event the impulse blocks in the HPS (no V), the tachycardia will terminate (see **Fig. 49**)[46] because ventricular activation is necessary for the AV-AP to be engaged. With antidromic (reverse of orthodromic) AV reentry, ipsilateral retrograde BBB prolongs the VA interval owing to HPS delay (**Fig. 53**).[64] In this scenario, retrograde conduction to the AV node and atrium will be delayed, and the CL of tachycardia will prolong. When the accommodation or migration of retrograde HPS block occurs, ipsilateral BB resumes conduction, VH (and consequently VA) shortens, and there is acceleration of tachycardia rate (see **Fig. 53**). Compared with retrograde conduction via ipsilateral versus contralateral BB conduction the tachycardia CL accelerates by 45 ms in **Fig. 53**. For AV-AP, which can insert into the left or RV freewall location, ipsilateral retrograde BBB can influence the tachycardia CL. With slow conduction AP (such as atriofascicular), which primarily occurs on the right side (with rare exception), only the RBBB (above the insertion of the AP in the RB) will influence CL (**Fig. 54**).[65,66]

Atrial pacing in patients with AV-AP and maximum ventricular preexcitation the HPS is engaged first retrograde (ie, before anterograde) and may have retrograde conduction delay and/or block along the ipsilateral BB. This can be shown with simultaneous recording of the HB and RB (**Fig. 55**). The activation of both potentials at the same time can only occur via the contralateral BB with subsequent retrograde conduction through the AV node (see **Fig. 54**).[65,66] So the so-called double ventricular response to A_2 is presumed to be via the AP and the NP, respectively. In fact, the HPS is being activated retrograde by the preexcited QRS. This is because if the impulse travels anterograde through the NP the H-RB activation sequence is similar to sinus rhythm, that is, H followed by RB potential, and not simultaneously (see **Fig. 55**). The subsequent atrial depolarization is via the AV node and various scenarios can emerge, and some are depicted in **Fig. 55**. The impulse can travel down ipsilateral BB, then transseptally and create a BBR (**Fig. 55**). So instead of the so-called double response to a single atrial extra stimulus, the circuit in fact is atrial-induced V_2 complex is fully preexcited and the next complex (V_3) is BBR of the physiologic nature and may terminate in the LBB or proceed to retrograde activate HB and continue the BBR via the RBB. An alternate interpretation may be that retrograde H results in retrograde AV nodal (HA) conduction, activates the atria, and then reaches the RV via the AP, that is, antidromic AV reentry. The strength of this argument is that atrial activation always precedes V activation. However, the A-A preceding the last V-V is significantly longer, but the H-H before the V-V maintains the same relationship. On the other hand, the initial slurring in each QRS complex of the QRS suggests the onset of ventricular activation via an AP, unlike the rapid onset of the QRS in BBR owing to HPS-V conduction. However, the shortening of the AV-V interval during the last two QRS complexes may be related to AV nodal dual pathways (short Ar to long Ar) leading to different input site into the RV and hence Ar-V shortening (**Fig. 55**).

There is always some confusion about the distinction between antidromic AV reentry versus AV nodal reentry incidental or bystander AP participation creating a different type of preexcited tachycardia. Several relatively unsatisfactory indirect criteria have been offered in the past. Actually, the issue can be resolved easily with additional BB recordings. If the preexcited tachycardia is AV nodal reentry the HB deflection will precede the BB potential, whereas it will be the reverse during antidromic AV reentrant tachycardia (see **Fig. 56**). Another interesting finding with AV nodal reentry and bystander ventricular preexcitation is no change in tachycardia CL with or without preexcitation (**Fig. 57**). The HV interval is prolonged, but shortens as soon as the preexcitation is abolished (see **Fig. 56**). This apparent or pseudo-prolongation of HV interval is because the H is not producing the subsequent QRS. It is the conduction to the atrium, that is, HA interval followed by an AV interval through the AP to produce preexcitation (H-A-V sequence) and hence the pseudo-HV prolongation. This is an important finding to distinguish antidromic AV reentry versus AV nodal reentry and bystander AP participation. This type of fully preexcited tachycardia (no exceptions) can only be sustained if there is linking in the HPS between the AV node impulse exiting and retrograde HPS excitation via the AP. A link of these 2 impulses in the AV node will terminate the AV nodal reentry and in the ventricle will create a fusion QRS complex.

The most common mechanism for orthodromic tachycardia initiation with ventricular pacing is block of V_2 or V_3 in the HPS (**Figs. 58** and **59**). The reason is relatively straightforward: if the V_2 impulse reaches the AV node (via retrograde H_2) and something also depolarizes the atria via the AP the atrial impulse cannot get through the AV node owing to prior penetration (concealed conduction) and hence cannot initiate orthodromic tachycardia. With a block of V_2 in the HPS, the same impulse reaches the atria via AP and then engages the AV node and conducts, encountering no AV nodal conduction delay and start orthodromic tachycardia. On the other hand, if V_2 produces an H_2 impulse will not find the AV node fully recovered. However, if H_2 is followed by V_3 owing to BBR, which in turn blocks retrograde in the HPS, the same scenario will take place as with V_2. The result will be the initiation of orthodromic SVT, the atrial impulse reaching the atrium by way of the AP (**Figs. 59** and **60**).

With RV pacing at the onset of orthodromic AVR, LBBB aberrancy may be noted because while V2 blocks in the LBB later than RBB and hence less recovered when the next atrial impulse arrives via AP. There is a common perception that SVT will have an LBBB pattern more likely when right ventricle is paced as it blocks retrograde in LBB later and hence still refractory to when anterograde impulse arrives. This is true primarily with retrograde functioning AP (**Fig. 59**). In the case of AV nodal reentry or atrial tachycardias this is less likely because if V_2 does not reach the AV node owing to block in the HPS it cannot initiate AV nodal reentry or atrial tachycardia unless AP coexists as discussed. In the event the V_2 does reach the AV node and initiates AV nodal reentry, it will then have to activate the HB the second time. Single V_2 followed by 2 successive HB activations (ie, retrograde H_2 and thenant H), when the impulse reaches the LBB, it is more than likely to have recovered excitability and hence likely to conduct normally.

In the case of AV nodal reentry or atrial tachycardias anterograde BBB and/or HPS block have no effect on the atrial rate of tachycardia, but can change the ventricular rate and QRS morphology owing to HPS conduction delay and block, creating interesting ECG patterns. Some of these are displayed in **Figs. 61** and **62**. The following phenomenon can be observed in these tracings: AV nodal reentry (slow-fast) with no change in the atrial CL regardless of BBB (right or left), BBH (no QRS), HPS WP, 2:1 block in the HPS and 1:1 P-QRS complex with BBB and narrow QRS during the SVT. See further details in the legend.

SUMMARY

In this article, many of the arrhythmias arising in an abnormal HPS are discussed, which is either the primary culprit or is intimately involved. Among the nontachycardia situations, BBB with its various manifestations is discussed. Also included are first-, second-, and third-degree AV block in the HPS and the current diagnostic criteria. A higher degree of block such as 2:1, 3:1, and intermittent second-degree block and some issues regarding their definition are also discussed.

Additionally, junctional premature complexes, automatic junctional tachycardia, idiopathic left posterior inferior fascicular tachycardia, and multiform left post inferior fascicular tachycardia are presented. There is a great deal of attention given to BB reentry, its underlying substrate, and at least the suggestion that this is the most common sustained form of VT among the HPS-related tachycardias. Furthermore its consequences are devastating if not properly diagnosed and treated because many of these patients have poor LVEF. In certain substrates, such as idiopathic cardiomyopathy, valvular disease, and muscular dystrophy, this form of tachycardia is particularly common. In all of these conditions the incidence exceeds 25% of the monomorphic VT diagnosed.

The role of the HPS in the setting of SVT and AP is also presented. The HPS affects the rate of these tachycardias, and many times initiation and termination is also affected. This is the case in particular in patients with overt or concealed AP because the ventricular myocardium is a part of the circuit and the HPS (orthodromic or antidromic). In other supraventricular tachycardia a change in HV interval or BBB can create complex ECG patterns. As mentioned in the introduction and worth repeating, it is critical to record additional potentials from BBs, which will make the diagnosis much easier. Without it, the chances of complex arrhythmia misinterpretation is greater.

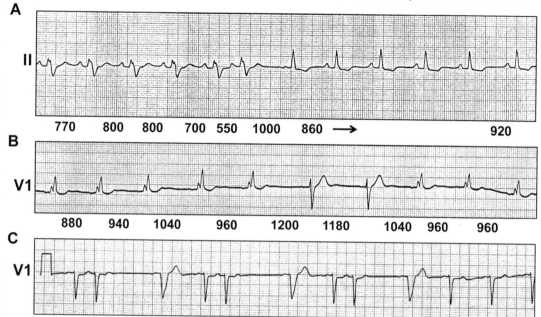

Fig. 1. Rate-related bundle branch block (phases III and IV). (*A*) Left bundle branch block (LBBB) pattern and (*B*) right bundle branch block (RBBB) pattern. During sinus rhythm, a single atrial premature complex slows the rate and the LBBB pattern disappears. A slight change of sinus rhythm, that is, slowing abolishes the RBBB (*B*). The measurements are in milliseconds. (*C*) Atrial bigeminy and the return cycle conducts with LBBB. When the pause is not long enough, the QRS is narrow (*last 3 complexes*).

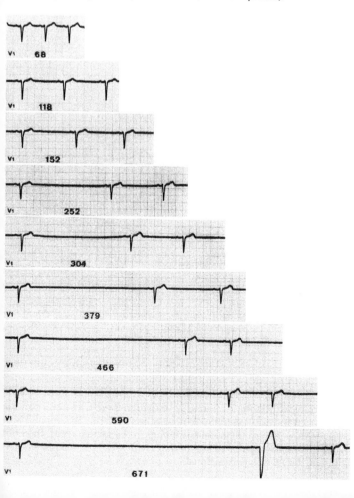

Fig. 2. Bradycardia phase IV bundle branch block. This figure is reproduced from Rosenbaum and colleagues in a clinical setting. It is clear that the progressive longer escape from the top panels is insufficient to manifest the phase IV block. In the last panel, note that there is a pause of 6.7 seconds before this type of block appears in this individual. (*From* Rosenbaum MB, Lazzari JO, Elizari MV. The Role of Phase 3 and Phase 4 Block in Clinical Electrocardiography. In: Wellens HJJ, Lie KI, Janse MJ, editors. The Conduction System of the Heart: Structure, Function and Clinical Implications. Leiden, the Netherlands: HE Stenfert Kroese; 1976: 126–42; page 129; with permission.)

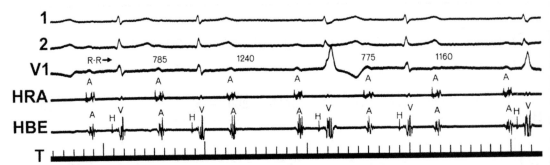

Fig. 3. Phase IV block in the His-Purkinje system. During atrioventricular nodal Wenckebach phenomenon, the first conducted complex shows a right bundle branch block pattern, whereas at faster rates, the QRS shows minimal abnormality.

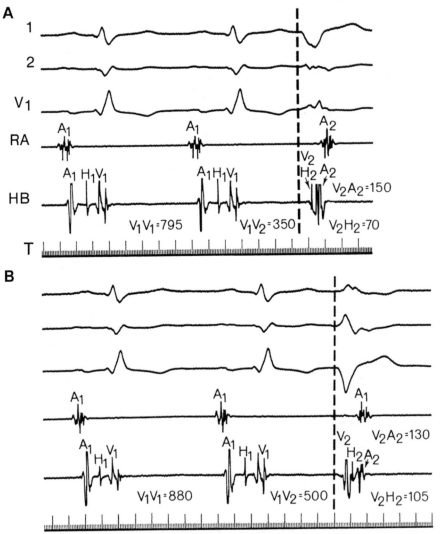

Fig. 4. Bidirectional block in right bundle branch block (RBBB). (*A*) During sinus rhythm there is an RBBB pattern. A single premature ventricular complex arises from the outflow (RBBB plus *right axis pattern*). The impulse activates the H_2 via the left bundle branch block ($V_2H_2 = 70$ ms). (*B*) In similar settings in the same patient, the right ventricular premature ventricular complex, V_2 even at a longer coupling conducts with a V_2H_2 of 105 ms, which is 45 ms longer compared with A, suggesting that the RBBB is bidirectional.

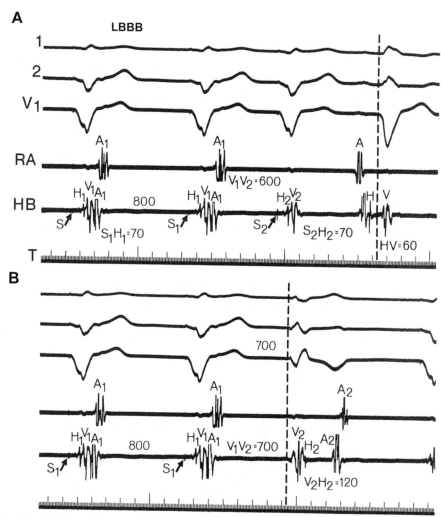

Fig. 5. Bidirectional block in left bundle branch block (LBBB). During sinus rhythm in the last QRS in (*A*), the patient has LBBB and normal axis. During right ventricular pacing at a basic CL of 600 ms, the retrograde H_1 and H_2 are activated via the right bundle branch. A single ventricular premature complex comes from the left ventricle (*B*; RBBB pattern); the retrograde H_2 now occurs via the contralateral bundle, that is, the right bundle, because the left bundle branch has a bidirectional block. The S_2H_2 in (*A*) is 70 ms whereas in (*B*) ie, V_2H_2 is 120, a 50 ms difference, which equates to transseptal conduction time.

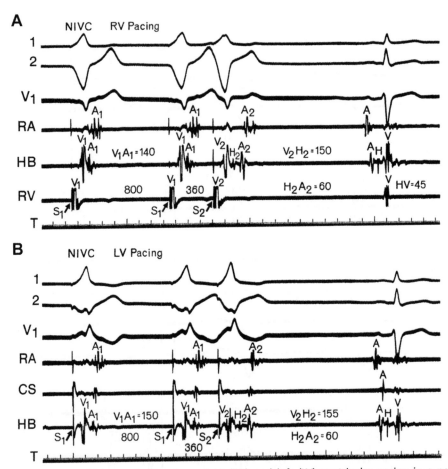

Fig. 6. Retrograde His-Purkinje conduction from right (RV) and left (LV) ventricular pacing in a patient with normal intraventricular conduction (NIVC). In the same patient, the retrograde His-Purkinje system V_2H_2 at identical coupling interval measures almost the same, that is 150 ms in (*A*) and 155 ms in (*B*; fairly comparable) and so is the atrioventricular nodal conduction at 60 ms. RA, right atrial.

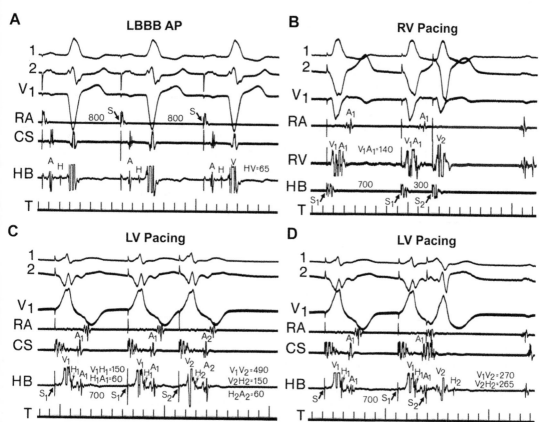

Fig. 7. Bidirectional block in left bundle branch block (LBBB). The LBBB pattern is seen in (*A*) during atrial pacing (AP) and there is slight prolongation of the HV interval, which is 65 ms. During right ventricular (RV) pacing (*B*). The V_1A_1 conduction is intact and shorter V_1V_2 interval blocks V_2 retrograde in the right bundle and subsequently in the left bundle and cannot reach the H_2. When the left ventricle is paced (*C*), the V_1H_1 is longer and the retrograde H_1 is visible during the basic drive, unlike in (*B*), and V_2 also conducts to the His and the atrium because in this case, the impulse travels transseptally to H_2 via the right bundle, which has intact conduction. (*D*) Block of V_2 above H_2, ie, the AV node. LV, left ventricular.

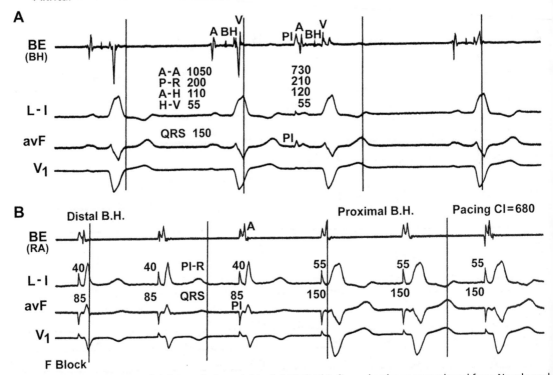

Fig. 8. (*A, B*) Site of lesion with left bundle branch block (LBBB). This figure has been reproduced from Narula and shows pacing from proximal and distal bundle of His (BH) in a patient who has LBBB and left axis deviation during sinus rhythm with proximal pacing of the His the QRS complex and axis remain the same as in sinus rhythm. A few millimeters distal to the original site of pacing, both the QRS and the axis completely normalize (*B*). The stimulus to the V interval corresponds to the HV intervals in both of these situations. All the pertinent intervals are labeled. (*From* Narula OS. Longitudinal dissociation in the His bundle. Bundle branch block due to asynchronous conduction within the His bundle in man. Circulation 1977;56:1001; with permission.)

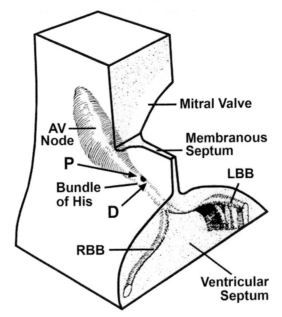

Fig. 9. Site of pacing in the left bundle (schematic). The schema presents the sites both proximal and distal of the His bundle and it is relatively close. The explanation of the results are in the text, which was cited as longitudinal dissociation of the His bundle. AV, atrioventricular; D, distal; LBB, left bundle branch; P, proximal; RBB, right bundle branch. (*From* Narula OS. Longitudinal dissociation in the His bundle. Bundle branch block due to asynchronous conduction within the His bundle in man. Circulation 1977;56:1004; with permission.)

Pacing Proximal to the Lesion (>>>)

Pacing Distal to the Lesion (>>>)

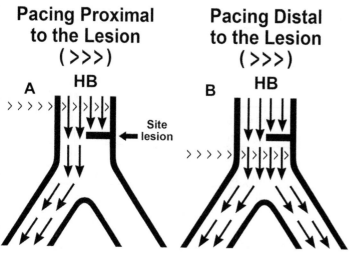

Longitudinal Dissociation

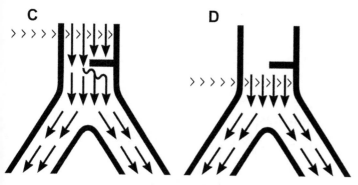

Anisotropic Conduction

Fig. 10. Anisotropic conduction. The purpose of this figure is to provide an alternate explanation for the findings in **Fig. 8**. The pacing sites are the same in *A* and *C*, and in *B* and *D*. The pacing site distally activates the entire His bundle (HB) with further longitudinal conduction along both bundles to normalize the QRS (*C, D*).

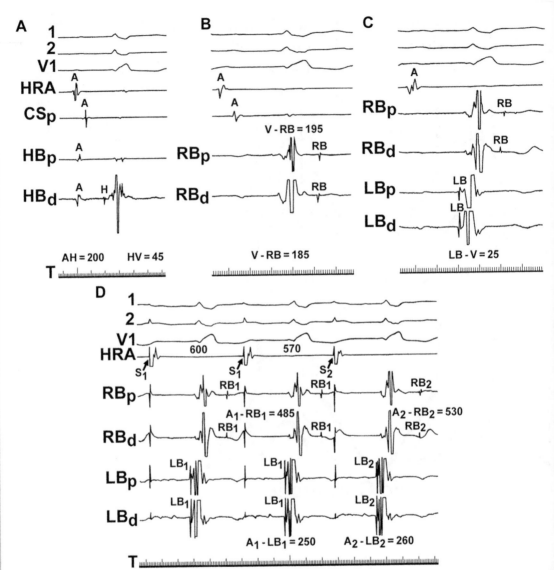

Fig. 11. Proximal delay in a patient with right bundle branch block (RBBB). (A–C) Sinus rhythm. The AH, HV, VRB, and LBV are labeled. As one can appreciate, RB recordings were added in B and LB in C. During sinus rhythm, the HV is normal and followed by transseptal conduction and then retrograde activation of the right bundle branch (ie, distal RB precedes proximal). This profound delay between the LB and RB through the septum can be further prolonged as shown with a relatively late atrial premature complex in D. (*Adapted from* Jazayeri M, Deshpande S, Sra J, et al. Retrograde (Transseptal) activation of right bundle branch during sinus rhythm. J Cardiovasc Electrophysiol 1993;4:281–4; with permission.)

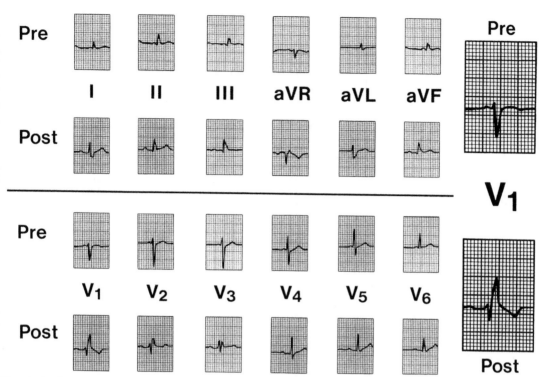

Fig. 12. Surface electrocardiographic (ECG) changes with right bundle ablation. The next three **Figs. 12–14** show that profound changes can occur following right bundle ablation in patients with His-Purkinje system disease. The patient had a normal ECG at baseline and normal HV intervals. Right bundle branch ablation resulted in traditional right bundle branch block with no additional abnormalities. **Figs. 13** and **14** are taken from patients with His-Purkinje disease.

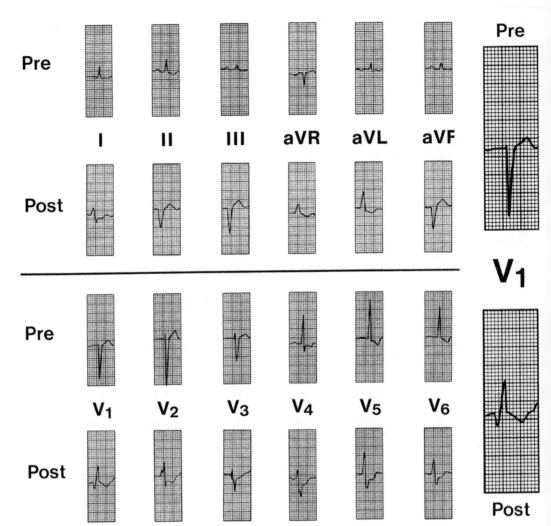

Fig. 13. Right bundle branch ablation in His-Purkinje system disease. The baseline shows a nonspecific intraventricular conduction. Note that after ablation there is a new pathologic Q wave in V$_1$ and leftward axis shift. See text for more details.

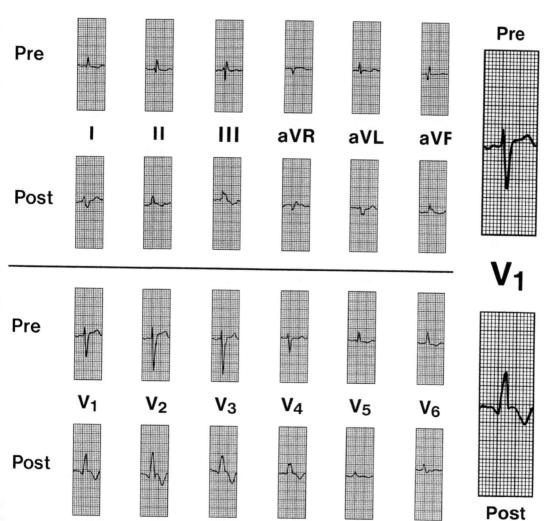

Fig. 14. Right bundle branch ablation in His-Purkinje system disease. The baseline electrocardiograph is normal except for some ST-T changes; the HV interval was prolonged. After ablation, there is a development of pathologic Q waves in V_1 and V_2 and rightward axis shift. See text for more details.

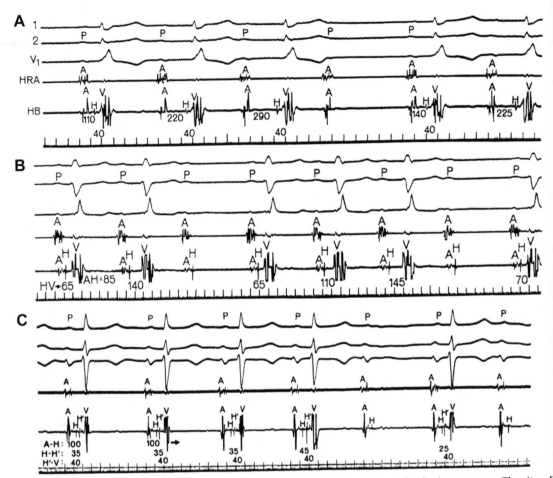

Fig. 15. Second-degree atrioventricular (AV) block. (*A–C*) Mobitz type I or Wenckebach phenomenon. The site of block in A is the AV node, infrahisian in B, and intrahisian in C. In all examples, there is progressive delay in the PR interval before the block. The example in C is subtle, where the 2 His deflections labeled H and H′ prolong only a few milliseconds before the block occurs after the first H.

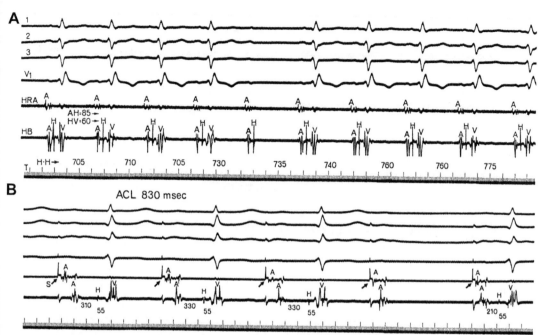

Fig. 16. Mobitz II AV block. The 2 panels are from different patients and show atrioventricular (AV) block with no PR prolongation before block. (*A*) Baseline electrocardiograph (ECG) showing right bundle, left axis, and the block below the His. (*B*) The QRS is normal and the key difference is the length of the PR interval, which is very long compared with A, whether this type of block is expected to occur in a patient with a long PR without much change before the block. If that is the case, the site of block and the ECG appearance of Mobitz II have a different meaning than what is traditionally seen in Mobitz II, ie, the site of block can be in the AV node unless the absolute length of PR interval is incorporated in the definition.

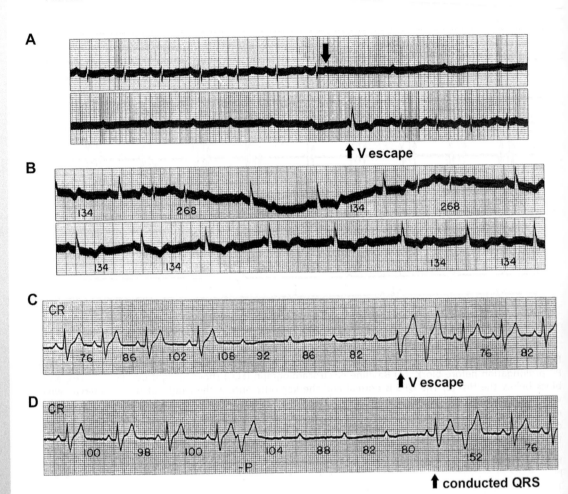

Fig. 17. Intermittent atrioventricular block. After a series of sinus complexes in *A*, a blocked atrial premature complex is followed by a series of p-waves without QRS until ventricular escape in the lower panel. (*B*) Idioventricular escape rhythm occasionally interspersed by a parasystolic focus, but the underlying rhythm is unaffected. (*C, D*) A series of blocked p-waves, either initiated by slight bradycardia (*C*) or a premature complex (*D*). The episodes end with ventricular escape (*C*) and conducted complex (*D*). See the text for more detail. (*Adapted from* Landgendorf R. Atrioventricular and intraventricular block. In: Langendorf R, Pick A, editors. Interpretation of complex arrhyhthmias. Philadelphia: Lea & Febiger (Springer); 1979. p. 346–50; with permission.)

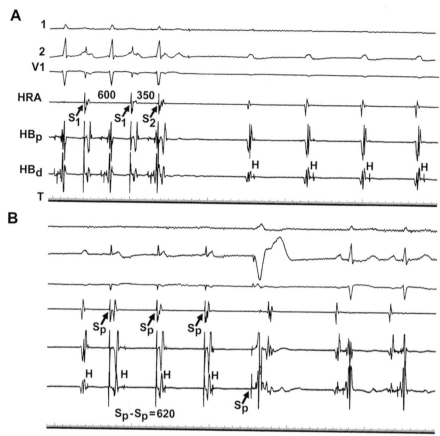

Fig. 18. Bradycardia-dependent atrioventricular (AV) block; A in this figure and A and B in **Fig. 17** suggest that bradycardia triggers this type of AV block because of spontaneous phase IV depolarization (hypopolarization). The episodes are often triggered by atrial or ventricular premature complexes. The duration of these episodes is unpredictable. In B, a ventricular premature complex also induces the resumption of AV conduction. The site of block is the His-Purkinje system.

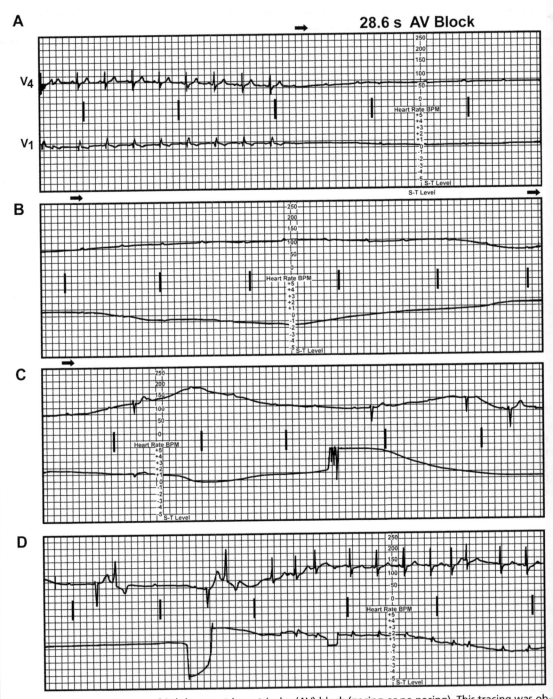

Fig. 19. (A, B) Second- versus third-degree atrioventricular (AV) block (pacing or no pacing). This tracing was obtained during sleep in an elderly female patient who had periodic symptoms of syncope but no documentation of the cause. The tracing starts with sinus rhythm and a right bundle branch block pattern and then a series of p-waves. There is no obvious trigger such as bradycardia or premature beats. The first detectable escape (C) occurs more than 28 seconds from the onset (D) shows resumption of AV conduction in the form of atrial fibrillation. The patient slept through the episode. This created many questions: (1) Is the episode better classified as second degree, high degree, or third degree? (2) Can it be vagal? (We have seen longer asystolic episodes owing to vaso-vagal episodes and managed without pacemakers.) (3) Can this episode be considered as asymptomatic? (4) Should the site of block be confirmed before permanent pacing? This patient refused electrophysiologic evaluation and required quite a bit of convincing to accept the pacemaker.

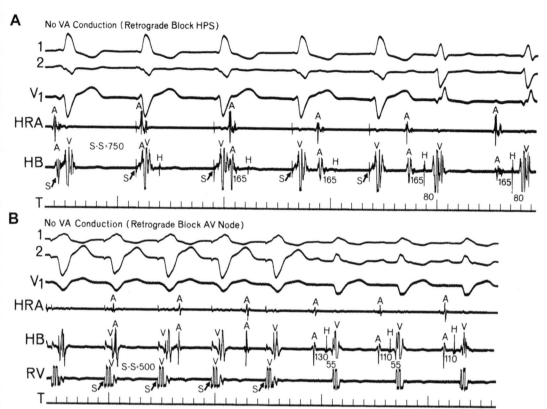

Fig. 20. Complete retrograde His-Purkinje system (HPS) block. The patient with bifascicular block (*A*) and long PR interval (both prolonged AH and HV) yet conducting 1:1 in the anterograde direction. No higher degree of atrioventricular (AV) block was documented, although he had some lightheaded spells. Several HPS abnormalities were found during electrophysiologic evaluation, that is, prolonged HV at 80 ms (trifascicular block) and complete retrograde HPS block. Note that the dissociated A blocked anterogradely below the His, whereas the AV nodal conduction remains constant at 165 ms during sinus rhythm (retrograde concealed conduction in the HPS). In contrast, *B* shows retrograde concealed conduction in the AV node. The dissociated sinus A waves all show delay or block in the AV node during ventricular pacing.

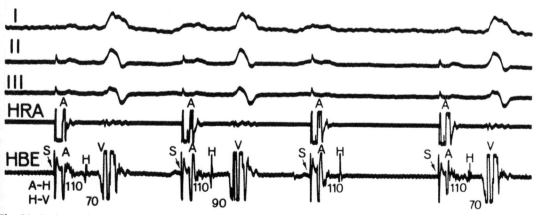

Fig. 21. Pacing-induced Wenckebach phenomenon (WP) in the His-Purkinje system (HPS). This patient was suspected of having HPS block but showed 1:1 conduction during sinus rhythm. Atrial pacing shows WP in the HPS, that is HV interval goes from 70 to 90 and then blocks. The HV is abnormal to begin with. This response suggests the need for a permanent pacemaker.

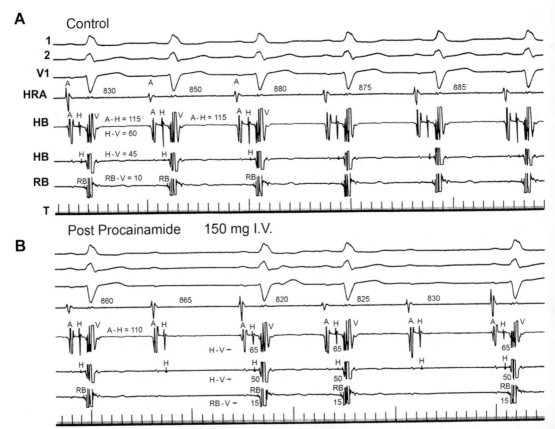

Fig. 22. Pharmaceutical stress on His-Purkinje system (HPS) conduction. (*A*) Sinus rhythm with a left bundle branch block, but 1:1 conduction. HV is slightly prolonged at 60 ms. (*B*) A small amount of intravenous procainamide (150 mg total) is injected. There are 2 His bundle and 1 right bundle recordings. At the baseline HRB interval is 50 ms from proximal His bundle as a result of pharmaceutical agent the conduction changes to 3:2 and 2:1 block in the HPS conduction. The site of block is between the His bundle and right bundle recording and hence fairly proximal. For conducted beats, the RBV interval after procainamide prolongs, which is the usual site of delay in the HPS after procainamide.

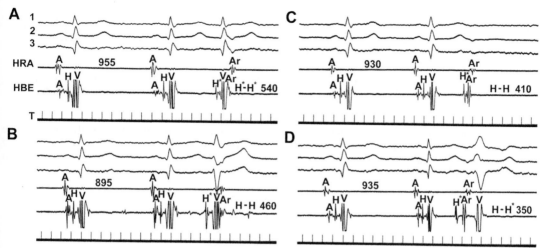

Fig. 23. Isolated junction extrasystole. (*A–D*) The first 2 complexes are sinus. After that, there are 4 junctional premature complexes (H*) with a different manifestation-based on H-H* coupling in each panel. (*A, B*) The H* conducts to the ventricle as well as to the atria. In A, the H_2 produces incomplete right bundle branch block pattern K. In B, the QRS shows left anterior superior fascicle. Following the H* (*C*) with shorter coupling interval the H_4 blocks toward the ventricle (no QRS) but produces a retrograde p-wave. Note the brevity of the p-wave compared with the sinus p-wave because the retrograde impulse exits toward in both atria simultaneously; therefore, it takes one-half the time. A fairly common observation from impulses originating at the atrioventricular node. (*D*) At even a shorter coupling interval, the anterograde conduction resumes with a long H* to V (gap phenomenon) and also conducts retrograde to the atria. Of particular notice is that the H* to A interval is variable in various panels, suggesting that the origin of junctional beats either from different locations in the His bundle, or owing to the prematurity of H-H* coupling interval.

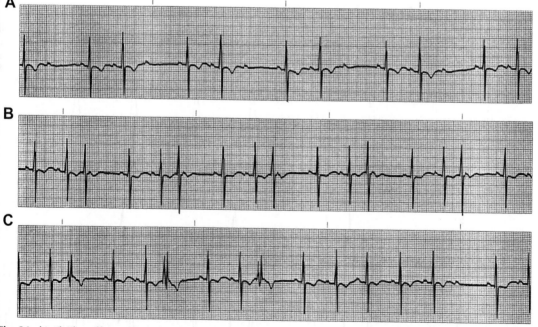

Fig. 24. (*A–C*) The effect of junctional premature complexes are shown. (*A*) The junctional beats block anterograde and retrograde but owing to atrioventricular (AV) nodal penetration, the next sinus p-wave, which is on time and blocks abruptly and unexpectedly, suggests a Mobitz type II AV block.[38] The junctional premature complexes reach the ventricle (*B*) and the sinus beat is seen at the end of the QRS the premature complex. The QRS of junctional origin is narrow in B and wide in C, which obscures the p-wave of sinus origin can barely be appreciated. However, in the same panel tracing, there is 1 p wave that blocks abruptly, as in A.

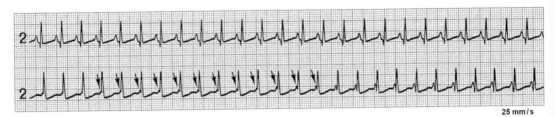

Fig. 25. Isoarrhythmic atrioventricular (AV) dissociation. This is an example where the sinus impulse can reach the ventricle (ie, there is no AV block); however, the junctional acceleration results in AV dissociation (*arrows*).[39] If sinus acceleration took place, or junctional pacemaker slows down, the AV conduction will resume as suggested in the top tracing.

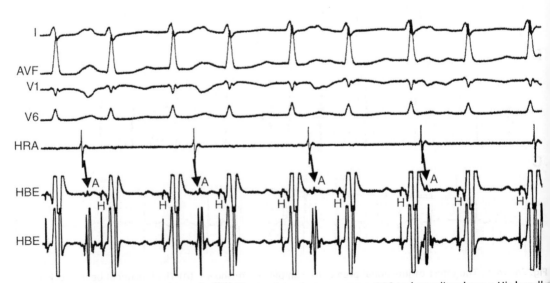

Fig. 26. Automatic junctional tachycardia.[40,41] The tracings show a narrow QRS tachycardia where a His bundle potential precedes all QRS complexes but no relationship between P and QRS complexes suggesting atrioventricular (AV) dissociation rather than the 1:2 AV conduction seen in the next figure. See text for detail. (*From* Gillette PC, Garson A Jr, Porter CJ, et al. Junctional automatic ectopic tachycardia: new proposed treatment by transcatheter His bundle ablation. Am Heart J 1983;106(4 Pt 1):619–23; with permission.)

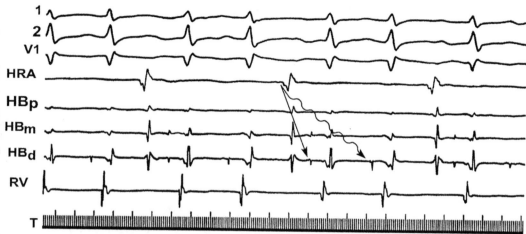

Fig. 27. A 1:2 atrioventricular (AV) response in a patient with dual AV nodal pathways.[42] The basic rhythm is sinus, but each sinus complex results in 2 QRS complexes, one through the fast pathway and next via the slow pathway. The conduction time through the fast pathway is not exactly 50% faster than the slow pathway; therefore, the RR intervals show a long short periodicity. Here the p-wave is conducting and hence it is an example of AV association not AV dissociation. The reason this AV nodal phenomenon is discussed here is because it is an important differential to what is seen in **Fig. 28**.

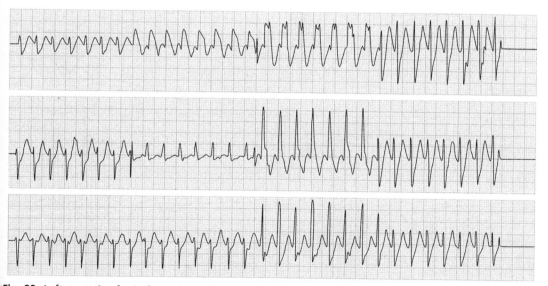

Fig. 28. Left posterior fascicular tachycardia. The 12-lead electrocardiograph of so-called verapamil-sensitive normal left ventricular tachycardia (VT) or left posterior fascicular tachycardia is shown. Two points are worth noting. (1) The initial deflection of the QRS is more rapid than traditionally seen with myocardial VT. (2) The left axis in this form of tachycardia is usually more leftward than left anterior superior fascicular block. This tachycardia frequently responds to intravenous verapamil and is not associated with any structural heart disease. See the text for more details.

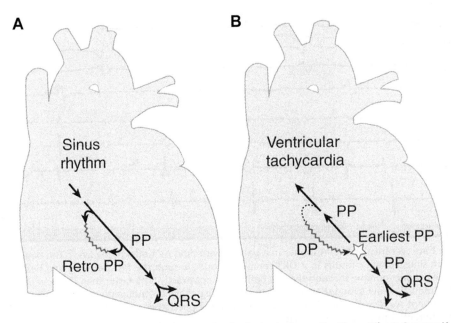

Fig. 29. (A, B) The proposed mechanism of left posterior fascicular tachycardia. (*From* Aiba T, Suyama K, Aihara N, et al. The role of Purkinje and pre-Purkinje potentials in the reentrant circuit of verapamil-sensitive idiopathic LV tachycardia. Pacing Clin Electrophysiol 2001;24:333–44; with permission.)

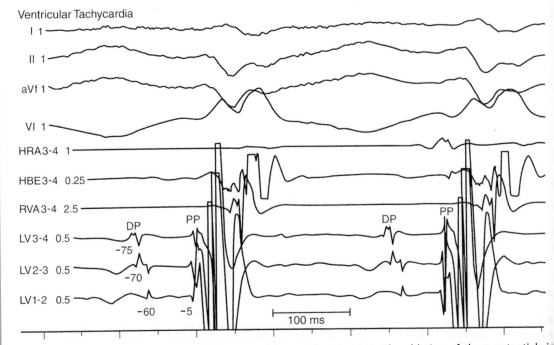

Fig. 30. Recording of diastolic and Purkinje potential preceding the QRS. The ablation of these potentials is frequently successful in eliminating tachycardia. (*From* Nogami A, Naito S, Tada H, et al. Demonstration of diastolic and presystolic Purkinje potentials as critical potentials in a macroreentry circuit of verapamil-sensitive idiopathic left ventricular tachycardia. J Am Coll Cardiol 2000;36:818; with permission.)

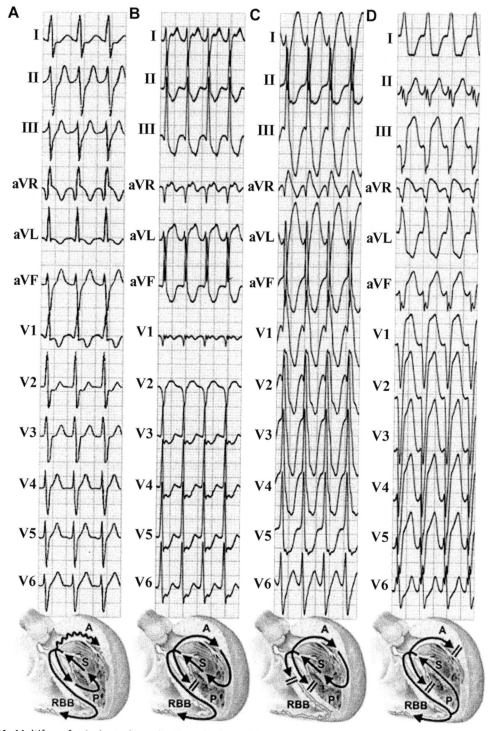

Fig. 31. Multiform fascicular tachycardia. Four displays of fascicular tachycardias are reproduced from **Fig. 24**. In *B*, the QRS is narrow and somewhat prolonged in *A*. The QRS is wide in *C* and *D*. (*C*) Right bundle and right axis morphology and (*D*) left bundle branch and left axis configuration. At the bottom of the tracing, the authors have shown a beautiful illustration through schematic. It should be noted that the septal division of the left bundle is only used in the retrograde direction. All of these tachycardias were ablatable with the exception of one, who needed long-term pharmacologic therapy. The usual successful site was at the base of the left bundle branch.

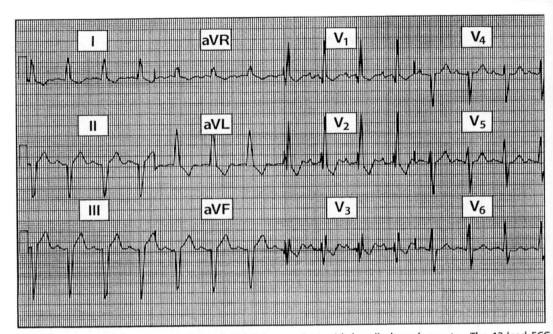

Fig. 32. Baseline 12-lead electrocardiograph (ECG) in a patient with bundle branch reentry. The 12-lead ECG shows sinus rhythm, normal PR interval, right bundle branch block, and left anterior superior divisional block. The patient has a history of syncope and although one could speculate that atrioventricular block is a possible underlying cause, the 2 forms of ventricular tachycardia that were induced in this patient are shown in **Fig. 33**.

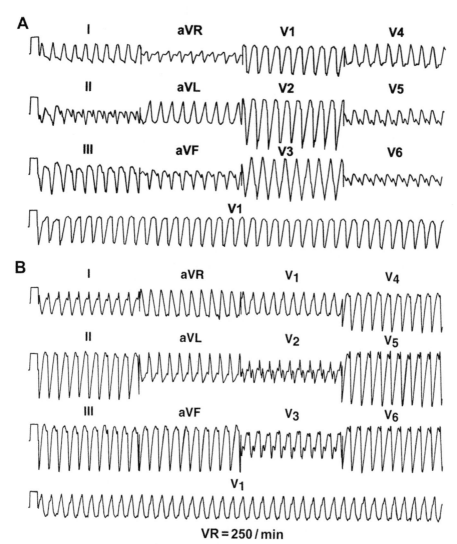

Fig. 33. Sustained bundle branch reentrant (BBR) tachycardia. These two 12-lead electrocardiographs (ECGs) are from the same patient whose baseline 12-lead ECG was shown in **Fig. 32**. Some observations are that (1) these are rapid ventricular tachycardias. (2) Both show a left axis deviation but somewhat different QRS configuration, that is, left (*A*) and right (*B*) bundle branch block pattern. (3) The left anterior superior divisional block is clear in B and suggestive in A. Despite a complete right bundle branch block pattern on surfaces ECG (**Fig. 32**) conduction intact bidirection conduction is, in fact, in the right bundle branch.

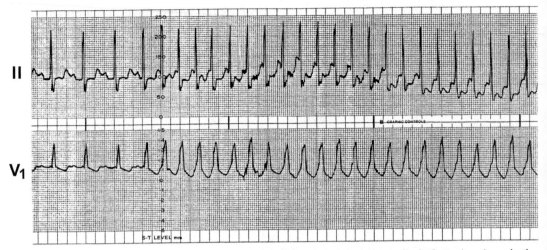

Fig. 34. Spontaneous onset of bundle branch reentrant (BBR) ventricular tachycardia (VT). During sinus rhythm, there is incomplete right bundle branch block (RBBB) and after 3 sinus complexes the VT starts. There is a shortening of the PR interval showing RBBB pattern with no change in prior RR intervals. Spontaneous initiation of VT without prior premature ventricular complex (myocardial or BBR) is the mechanism of VT onset in more than 75% of the cases. In other words, in spontaneous setting, VT, or for that matter BBR, is seldom triggered by premature beats. The underlying mechanism is aborted reentry that occurs in any reentry circuit, that is, the reentrant impulse is waiting to exit when the appropriate conditions are met. This is why the first QRS complex of the tachycardia has the same configuration as the remainder of the tachycardia. The alternative explanation that has been previously proposed—that is, that the initial complex is premature, which triggers the ensuing tachycardia (although both have QRS morphology that is identical), is a less convincing hypothesis.

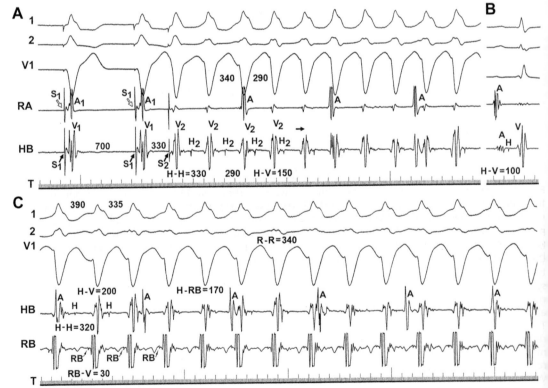

Fig. 35. Induction of sustained bundle branch reentrant (BBR) tachycardia. (*A*) The same patient as in **Fig. 34**. During stimulation of the right ventricle the tachycardia is initiated showing a left bundle branch block (LBBB) pattern. There is a reference sinus complex (*B*) with a prolonged HV interval and incomplete right bundle branch block pattern. Additional clues pointing to BBR include: (1) atrioventricular (AV) dissociation, (2) the HV interval is prolonged during the baseline and even longer during the tachycardia (150 vs 100 ms), and (3) LBBB morphology because it was initiated by right ventricular pacing.[40,41] (*C*) An RB recording is added and there is a long HRB interval (H - RB = 170 ms), suggesting conduction delay in the proximal His-Purkinje system, which in this case is owing to the underlining pathology which was aortic valve disease and its subsequent replacement. (4) The unusual degree of delay in the anterior limb, that is, the RBB, is in between the H and the RBB (*B*). RBB, right bundle branch recording

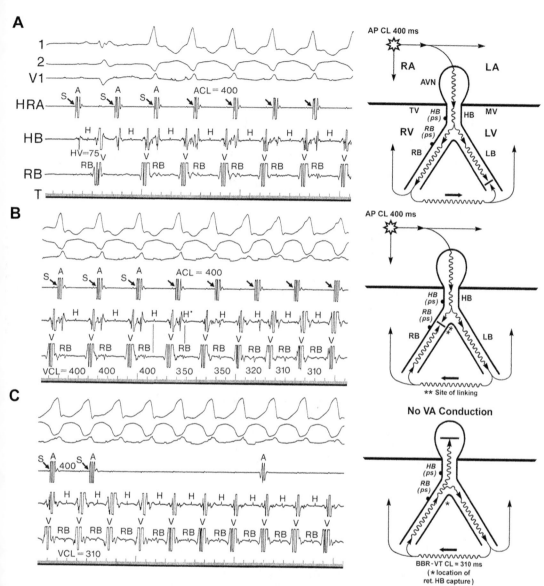

Fig. 36. Atrial induction of bundle branch reentrant (BBR) tachycardia. In all 3 panels (*A–C*), both right bundle branch and His bundle recordings are available. Atrial pacing at a CL of 400 ms is started in A. The first paced QRS complex has a long HV and a nonspecific intraventricular conduction defect of the left bundle branch block type. Because this patient has no accessory pathway, all the phenomenology is occurring within the His-Purkinje system. The second paced QRS results in farther prolongation of HV, but this time there is an RBBB pattern. The right bundle potential disappears from its earlier location, which occurred before the QRS in the first complex and moves to a location after the QRS during right bundle branch block, indicating its retrograde activation. The process continues where the His bundle (HB) is activated anterograde through the atrial impulse and the right bundle is depolarized by transseptal conduction in a retrograde fashion. This linking by interference ultimately breaks when there is retrograde capture of the HB via the RB (*indicated by an asterisk*). Bundle branch reentrant ventricular tachycardia and its corresponding RB-H sequence of bundle branch activation continues. When the atrial pacing is stopped in C, one can appreciate the ongoing BBR tachycardia (*from the point of asterisk*) without change in the RB-H sequence preceding the QRS and unrelated atrial activation. (*Adapted from* Caceres J, Jazayeri M, McKinnie J, et al. Sustained bundle branch reentry as a mechanism of clinical tachycardia. Circulation 1989;79:261; with permission.)

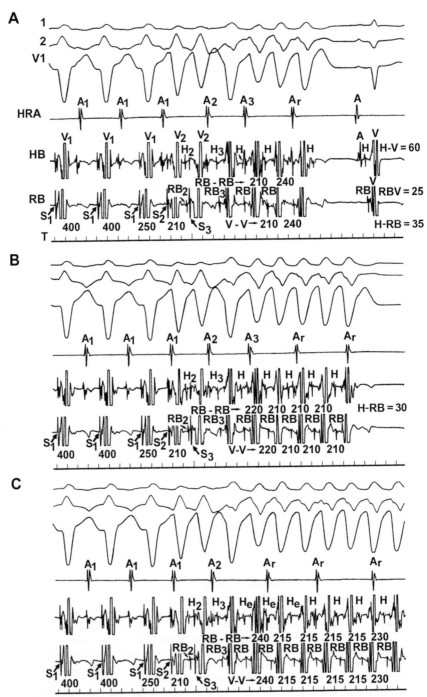

Fig. 37. Bundle branch reentrant (BBR) tachycardia and His-Purkinje system block. All panels show induction of BBR ventricular tachycardia (VT) with ventricular pacing displaying a left bundle branch block and left axis deviation pattern, different than the paced complexes. Nonetheless, some aspects are worth noting: (1) The baseline HV is prolonged and the H-RB is equal to 35 ms (*sinus complex*). (2) (*A*) Spontaneous termination of the VT takes place when the His bundle (HB) potential is not followed by RB potential, that is, block in the anterior limb (between the HB and the RB). (3) (*B*) Spontaneous termination occurs in the retrograde limb, that is, no H after the last QRS. (4) The H-RB during BBR measures 30 ms, indicating retrograde HB activation via the LBB. (5) Continuous sustained BBR (*C*) without termination with 2:1 VA block. (*From* Caceres J, Jazayeri M, McKinnie J, et al. Sustained bundle branch reentry as a mechanism of clinical tachycardia. Circulation 1989;79:266; with permission.)

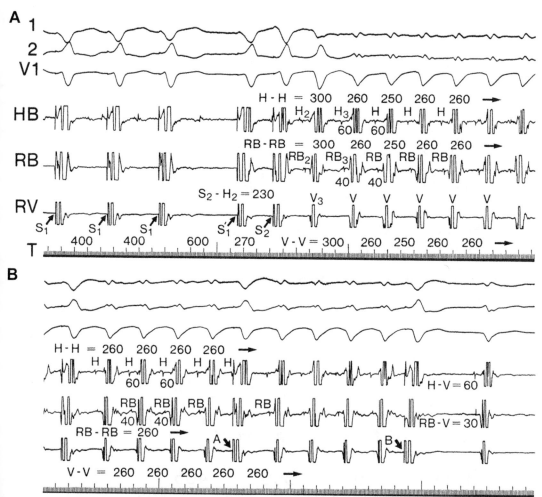

Fig. 38. Bundle branch reentrant (BBR) tachycardia and the effect of programmed ventricular extrastimuli. (*A*) The BBR is triggered with the pacing protocol, which uses a short–long–short sequence that has been in our experience more effective in initiating this form of reentry, and even in many cases, myocardial ventricular tachycardia. The HRB is 20 ms versus 30 ms during baseline rhythm (*last complex in B*), suggesting activation of the His bundle (HB) retrograde via the left bundle branch. An attempt is made to terminate the tachycardia (*B*). The first ventricular premature complex manages to capture the HB and the tachycardia is simply reset. The next premature complex blocks retrograde in the His-Purkinje system and terminates the BBR. (*From* Caceres J, Jazayeri M, McKinnie J, et al. Sustained bundle branch reentry as a mechanism of clinical tachycardia. Circulation 1989;79:265; with permission.)

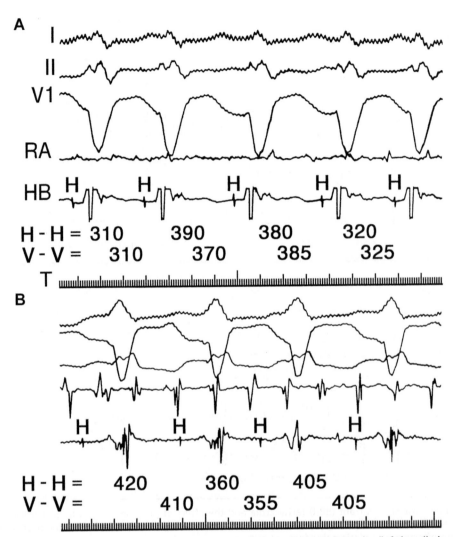

Fig. 39. H-H and V-V relationships during bundle branch reentrant (BBR) tachycardia (left bundle branch block configuration in *A* and right bundle branch block in *B*). One of the characteristics and important aspects to find the driver of the arrhythmia. In the case of BBR, it is important to determine whether H-H is driving the V-V or the reverse. This figure shows both right and left bundle branch block pattern of BBR and significant variation in CL. It clearly demonstrates His bundle activation driving the ventricle and not the other way around.

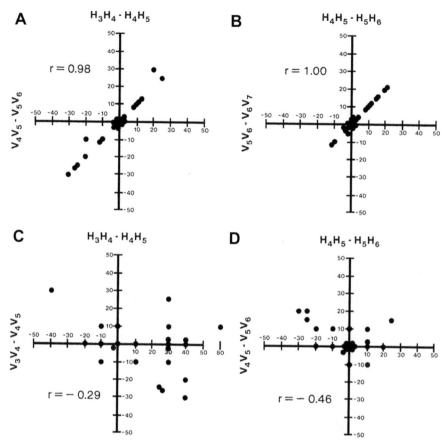

Fig. 40. H-H versus V-V CL relationship during bundle branch reentrant tachycardia. The concept presented here is now applied to many more patients. These relationships between preceding and subsequent events are plotted in the 4 scenarios shown. (*A, B*) It can be appreciated that there is an excellent correlation of His bundle activation with subsequent QRS and not the previous. The opposite is seen in *C* and *D*, where there is a wide scatter and no correlation. (*From* Caceres J, Jazayeri M, McKinnie J, et al. Sustained bundle branch reentry as a mechanism of clinical tachycardia. Circulation 1989;79:264; with permission.)

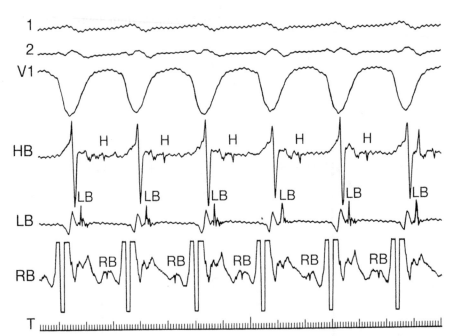

Fig. 41. H–RB–LB activation sequence preceding bundle branch reentrant tachycardia. The tachycardia configuration is left bundle branch block pattern and the expected reentry circuit would be His bundle (HB) activation through the left bundle branch (LBB) and then HB activates RB anterior and produces the QRS. After transseptal conduction, the LBB is activated in retrograde and the process continues H > RB > QRS > LB. Then the sequence is repeated.

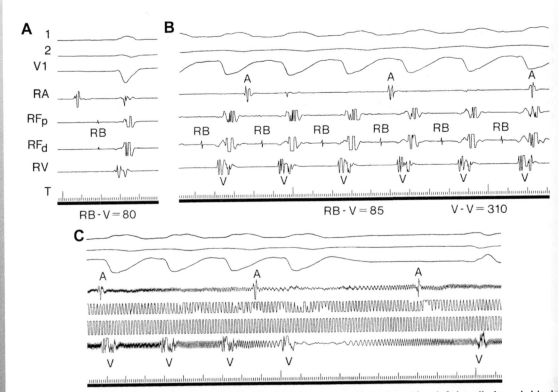

Fig. 42. Right bundle branch ablation in bundle branch reentrant tachycardia with a left bundle branch block (LBBB) pattern. Sinus rhythm complex (*A*) and bundle branch reentrant ventricular tachycardia (*B*) both show an LBBB pattern. The RBV intervals are labeled. The right bundle branch ablation terminates the tachycardia. Subsequent sinus complex shows a right bundle branch block. (*C*) It can also be appreciated that the PR interval of the sinus beat after ablation is longer than the PR before ablation.

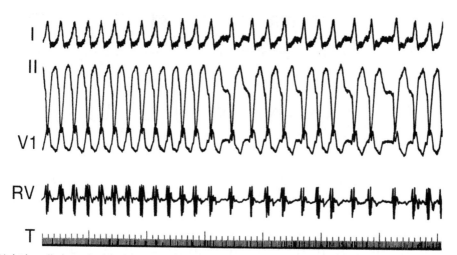

Fig. 43. Right bundle branch ablation in a bundle branch reentrant tachycardia with a right bundle branch block pattern. Ongoing bundle right branch reentry ventricular tachycardia showing right bundle and left axis morphology is regular seen in the first one-half of the tracing. Right bundle branch ablation is initiated, which terminates the tachycardia. The QRS morphology remains identical, but is now irregular because the underlying rhythm is now atrial fibrillation.

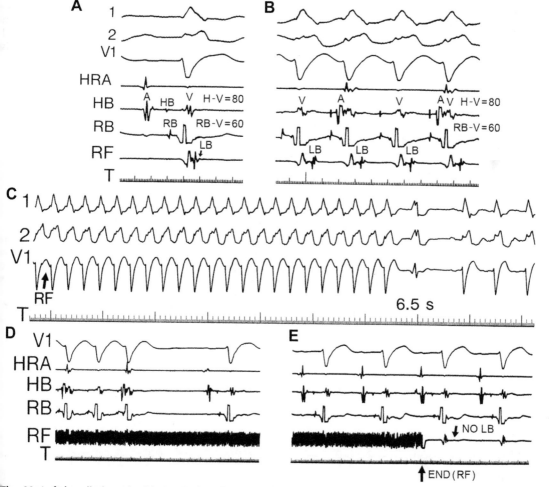

Fig. 44. Left bundle branch ablation in bundle branch reentrant (BBR) tachycardia with a left bundle branch block pattern. The sinus complex in *A* and BBR ventricular tachycardia in *B* are depicted along with His bundle (HB), RB, and LB recordings. (*C–E*) One can appreciate the sequence of events during sinus and tachycardia. His bundle activation is first followed by the right bundle and then the impulse transseptally activates the left bundle retrograde. The ablation eliminates the tachycardia and does not change the QRS, but the bundle branch potential (*arrow*) is no longer visible.

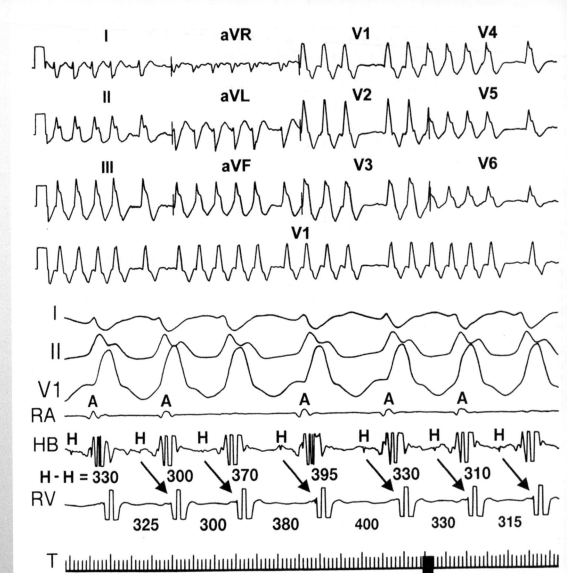

Fig. 45. Interfascicular reentry. This example is of a patient who had prior ablation of the right bundle branch owing to bundle branch reentrant tachycardia. However, the patient developed more frequent episodes, which at some point became incessant. This is depicted in the surface electrocardiograph (ECG) and with intercardiac signals. The ECG showed the morphology of right bundle branch block most likely owing to ablation and right axis and a normal PR interval. (*Adapted from* Blanck Z, Sra J, Akhtar M. Incessant interfascicular reentrant ventricular tachycardia as a result of catheter ablation of the right bundle branch: case report and review of the literature. J Cardiovasc Electrophysiol 2009:20:1280–1; with permission.)

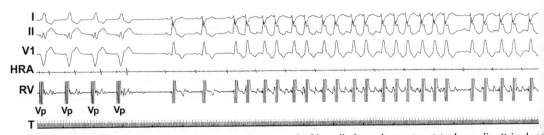

Fig. 46. The effect of right ventricular pacing on the control of bundle branch reentrant tachycardia. It is clear that during the pacing, which is shown in the initial part of the tracing, there is no ventricular tachycardia and a 1:1 pacing response. As soon as the pacing is stopped, after a couple of sinus cycles the patient goes back into incessant tachycardia identical to **Fig. 45**.

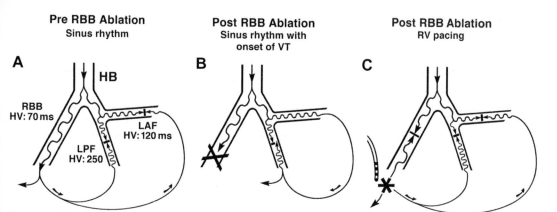

| Pre RBB Ablation | Post RBB Ablation | Post RBB Ablation |
| Sinus rhythm | Sinus rhythm with onset of VT | RV pacing |

A HB
RBB HV: 70 ms
LAF HV: 120 ms
LPF HV: 250

B

C

Fig. 47. Interfascicular reentry. The figure shows 3 schemas: (*A*) Pre right bundle branch ablation (RBB). (*B*) Post RBB ablation. (*C*) Post RBB ablation and right ventricular (RV) pacing. These schemas present the sequence of events that took place. (*A*) Before the first ablation with right bundle conduction intact and therefore the impulse transseptally invaded the left ventricle and prevented interfascicular reentry by partial penetration of the various divisions of the left bundle. When the right bundle was ablated, then this retrograde penetration of the left bundle branch divisions was no longer possible, and therefore the conduction delay already present in the anterior superior and posterior inferior divisions created a reentrant circuit with incidental bystander participation of the right bundle owing to ablation. (*B*) The route of impulse propagation was retrograde via the anterior superior division and then anterograde along the inferior posterior division, necessitating a fascicular ablation. The reason right ventricular pacing was effective in preventing the interfascicular Ev reentry was because it accomplished the same goal as was shown in A, that is, effective retrograde penetration of the various fascicles of the left bundle branch. (*From* Blanck Z, Sra J, Akhtar M. Incessant interfascicular reentrant ventricular tachycardia as a result of catheter ablation of the right bundle branch: case report and review of the literature. J Cardiovasc Electrophysiol 2009:20:1282; with permission.)

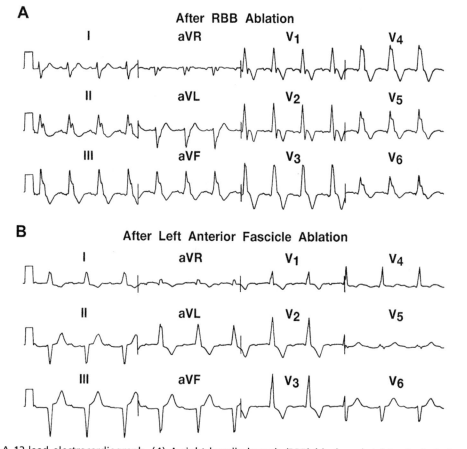

A   After RBB Ablation

I   aVR   V₁   V₄

II   aVL   V₂   V₅

III   aVF   V₃   V₆

B   After Left Anterior Fascicle Ablation

I   aVR   V₁   V₄

II   aVL   V₂   V₅

III   aVF   V₃   V₆

Fig. 48. A 12-lead electrocardiograph. (*A*) A right bundle branch (RBB) block and right axis deviation during which the patient was experiencing incessant tachycardia. (*B*) Additional ablation of left anterior fascicle, abolition of tachycardia, and a change in the QRS morphology somewhere, left axis shift, and a long PR interval. The patient no longer has interfascicular or bundle branch reentry.

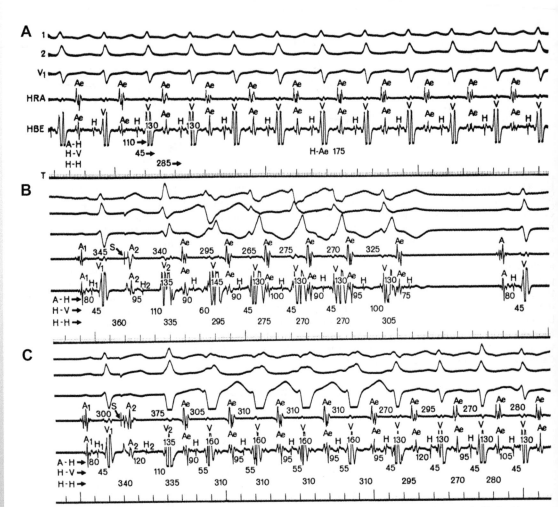

Fig. 49. Effect of the His-Purkinje system (HPS) on an accessory pathway. An example of concealed left side accessory pathway and the effect of HPS conduction delay and block is presented in this and the next **Figs. 50** and **51.** This patient has left freewall AP, which could be determined even though there is no coronary sinus recoding. (*A*) Orthodromic tachycardia with narrow QRS. The relevant intervals—A-H, H-V, and H-H—are labeled. (*B*) Aberrant conduction during which one can see a right bundle branch block (RBBB), minor left axis shift, a major left axis shift, and normal axis. The V-A interval labeled in the middle of the ventricular electrocardiograph measures 130 ms and during QRS complexes, which show RBBB and/or right axis because they will have no relevance to affect conduction in this particular AP. The difference between a right bundle and right bundle with left axis seen in B is 15 ms longer in the case of axis deviation. The final atrial complex is followed by a His bundle and no QRS and terminates the tachycardia. The further prolongation of VA interval to 160 ms is seen with complete left bundle branch block pattern in C and the CL changes when the aberrancy disappears. (*From* Akhtar M, Damato AN, Ruskin JN, et al. Anterograde and retrograde conduction characteristics in three patterns of paroxysmal atrioventricular junctional reentrant tachycardia. Am Heart J 1978:95:28; with permission.)

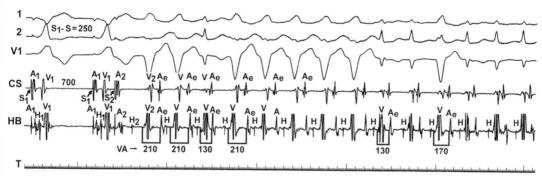

Fig. 50. Coronary sinus pacing in a patient with left freewall AP, atrial premature beat A_2 initiations the tachycardia with left bundle branch block, and left axis, which sometimes is normal (*4th complex from the end*). It can be noticed that the VA interval is 80 ms longer with left axis compared with narrow QRS and 40 ms longer compared with left bundle and normal axis.

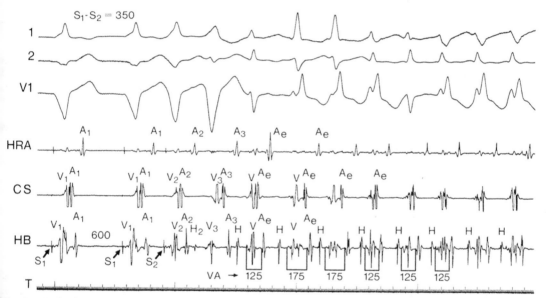

Fig. 51. Orthodromic tachycardia is initiated with ventricular premature stimulation and various QRS morphologies, which include left bundle left axis, right bundle and left axis, right bundle and normal axis, and right bundle and right axis, as well as 2 normal QRS complexes. It is remarkable that only the right bundle and left axis meaning only the left axis produces a VA prolongation aside from the paced beats themselves, which arise from the right ventricle.

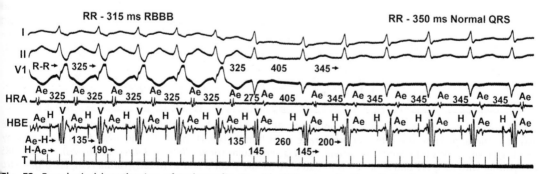

Fig. 52. Paradoxical lengthening of tachycardia CL with QRS normalization. Orthodromic tachycardia using a right freewall AP. In the middle of the tracing, there is normalization of the QRS, and consequent shortening of the AA cycle engages slow AV nodal pathway with a long AH of 260 ms. The rest of the tachycardia is therefore slower owing to the engagement of the slow pathway. The RR interval during right bundle branch block and during narrow QRS tachycardia is listed on top of lead I. All the other pertinent intervals are also labeled.

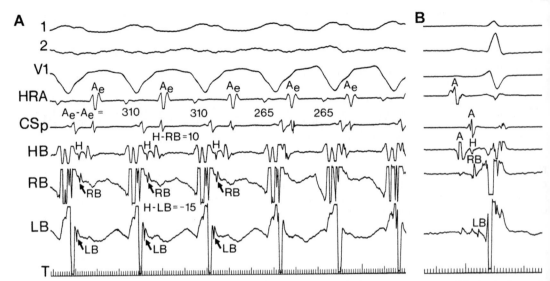

Fig. 53. Role of the His-Purkinje system (HPS) in antidromic atrioventricular reentry supraventricular tachycardia (SVT) using fast conduction AP. (*A*) Wide QRS tachycardia using a right-sided AP anterograde and normal pathway retrograde is shown. The sequence of retrograde HPS conduction comes after the QRS that is LB, RB, His bundle, and then the QRS. The His-Purkinje delay in the retrograde direction causes significant slowing of the SVT (CL of 310 ms). The abolition of retrograde block and merging of retrograde A into the ventricular electrogram and shortening of the CL from 310 to 265 ms can be noted in *B*. In B, simply shown is a reference sinus complex along with the intracardiac electrogram.

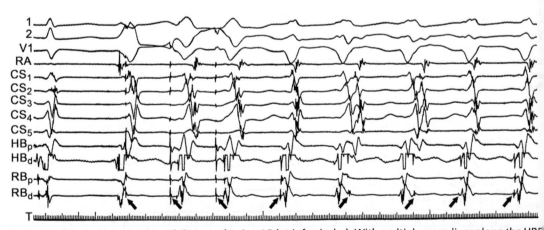

Fig. 54. The His-Purkinje system and slow conduction AP (atriofascicular). With multiple recordings along the HRB axis, one can appreciate the effect of retrograde right bundle branch block on the atrial fascicular pathway which typically inserts into the right bundle. After 3 ventricular stimuli (*leftward directed arrows*), a wide QRS tachycardia with long AV and short VA is initiated. After the second and third tachycardia complex (*rightward directed arrows*), the right bundle branch potential now follows the QRS and prolongs the VA time. It can also be appreciated that there is a separation of the VA potentials in coronary sinus 2 to 4 and proximal His (HB) bundle labeled HBp. The result of flowing of AA interval, which accelerates as soon as the ipsilateral bundle branch (right bundle branch) starts conducting normally (*the last 2 QRS complexes*). It should also be noted that the RB potential now receives the QRS, typical of atrial fascicular connection from the atrium to the right bundle

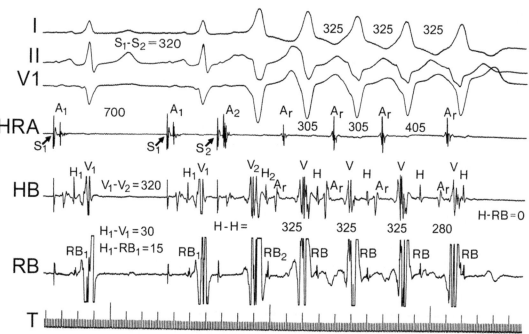

Fig. 55. Wide QRS tachycardia in a patient with ventricular preexcitation. At a basic CL of 700 ms, atrial pacing S_1S_1, A_1A_1, a single atrial premature complex (S_2, A_2) conducts with full preexcitation. This part of the figure was also shown in **Fig. 7**, with the difference being that now there is an additional right bundle recording and there is a wide QRS tachycardia. The A_2 in fact does not conduct via the atrioventricular (AV) node, but via the left bundle branch in retrograde. That is the reason the HRB interval shortens from 15 to 0 ms. A subsequent atrial activation is via the AV node labeled AR and not an AV nodal echo. The subsequent events have at least 2 different interpretations. (1) Antidromic AV reentry. (2) Bundle branch reentry and (3) AV nodal reentry with standby accessory pathway participation. The first possibility, that antidromic reentry has the sequence of AP > RV > LB > AV node > atrial activation supports this diagnosis. The patient does have what looks like a preexcited complex and each QRS is preceded by A. However, working against this possibility is that the last AA interval is markedly longer than the subsequent RR interval, that is, 405 versus 325 ms. This, however, can be explained by retrograde conduction switch from a fast to a slow pathway exiting closer to the atrial insertion. (2) In favor of bundle branch reentrant tachycardia is that the H_2H preceding the RR interval have identical duration of 325 ms. (3) The fact that the impulse is activating the His bundle via the left bundle and not turning around in the node excludes AV nodal reentry. RV, right ventricular.

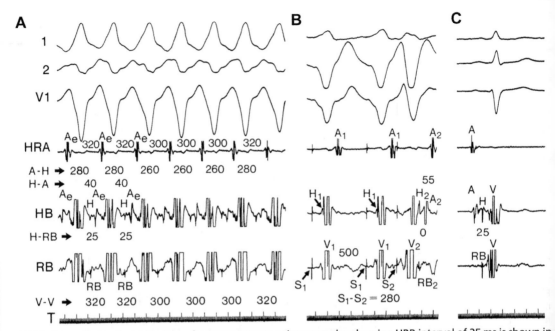

Fig. 56. Preexcited tachycardia. For reference purposes a sinus complex showing HRB interval of 25 ms is shown in C. (*B*) Retrograde activation of the His by shortening the RBV interval to 0. These 2 panels function as a reference to A, which shows a preexcited tachycardia, and the HRB sequence during the tachycardia is H followed by RB with an HRB interval of 25 ms. This could only happen if the impulse was coming from the atrioventricular node and rules out true antidromic reentry.

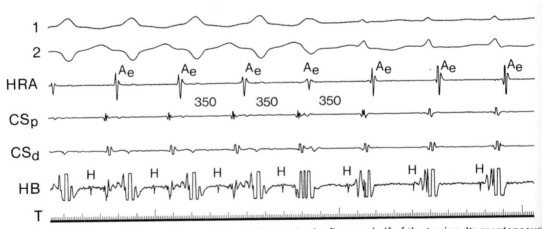

Fig. 57. Preexcited tachycardia. An unusual wide QRS is seen in the first one-half of the tracing. Its spontaneous premature ventricular complex changes the wide QRS to a narrow QRS tachycardia with the same CL. A very unusual phenomenon is also occurring, which involves the HV interval. During the tachycardia with a wide QRS there was a very long HV interval, which shortens to the normal HV interval as expected in atrioventricular (AV) nodal reentry. This is shown in the last part of the tracing. The explanation for this pseudo-HV prolongation during the wide QRS tachycardia is that atrial activation must occur before the QRS can be activated even as a bystander. So the sequence of H, A, and V gives the impression that the His is related to the subsequent QRS. In fact the H produces the A, which then creates preexcitation. Once that part of the process is eliminated—that is, preexcited, the underlying AV nodal reentry becomes manifest.

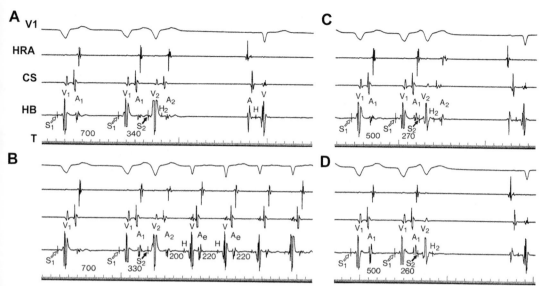

Fig. 58. Mechanism of atrioventricular (AV) reentry initiation with ventricular pacing. **Fig. 55** depicts what is required to initiate orthodromic reentry with right ventricular pacing. In all panels, the basic drive V_1V_1 is 700 ms and V_1V_2 is progressively decreased from A to D. (*A*) Retrograde activation of the His bundle via the normal pathway and atrial that is A_2 through the AP. In *B*, V_2 blocks in the His-Purkinje system (now A_2 precedes H) the A_2 activation is via the AP, which engages anterograde the AV node and initiates an orthodromic tachycardia with the coronary sinus electrogram preceding all the other electrograms, suggesting left-sided AP. Note also that the first AH, that is A_2H of 200 ms is shorter than the subsequent one. The return of H_2 in *C* abolishes orthodromic tachycardia induction, because now the A_2 reduced by the AP can no longer find the AV node recovered from anterograde conduction. In *D*, the V_2 blocks in the AP and also along the normal pathway, but in the AV node.

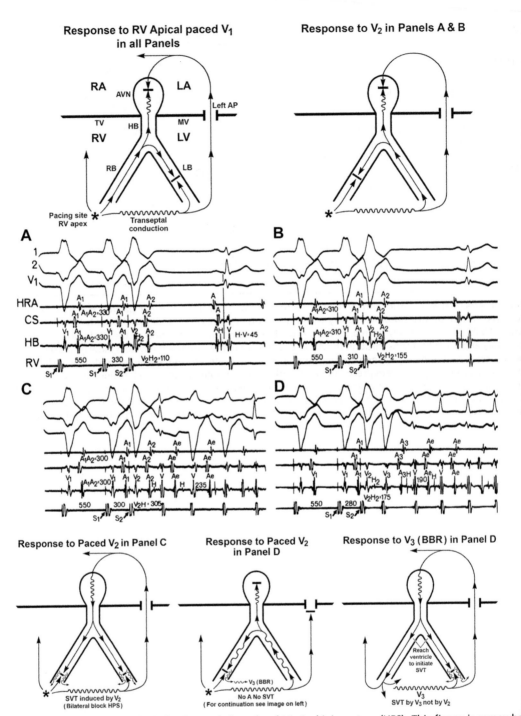

Fig. 59. Orthodromic tachycardia induction and the role of His-Purkinje system (HPS). This figure is somewhat similar to **Fig. 58**, particularly in *A* and *B*, which are also explained in the accompanying schema. In both of these panels, the retrograde His is activated through the normal pathway and the AP activation is independent of that. The atrial activation sequence, that is coronary sinus electrogram first, suggest left freewall AP. In *C*, V_2 blocks in the HPS and initiates the orthodromic reentry as happened in *B* of **Fig. 58**. When the H_2 returns as happens in D, there is also concomitant block in the AP, so there is no A_2. Because of the V_2H_2 delays, V_3 phenomenon (bundle branch reentrant tachycardia) occurs, which in turn blocks in the HPS and conducts to the atrium (A_3) to start the orthodromic tachycardia. The accompanying schematics can somewhat clarify what was just discussed.

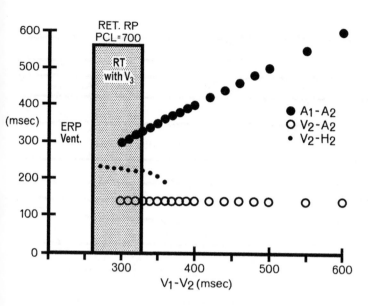

Fig. 60. Scanning of basic CL with V_1V_2 in patient with AP. The V_1V_2 in milliseconds are plotted against various other parameters the filled circles represent A_1, A_2; open circles represent V_1A_2 and the small black dots represent V_2H_2. During the scanning V_2A_2 intervals do not change. The A_1A_2 shows a typical curve that shortens as the V_1V_2 intervals decrease. The H emerges at about 360 ms, however, as long as the H is present there is no tachycardia. In the hatched area V_3, which blocks in the His-Purkinje system, initiates orthodromic tachycardia.

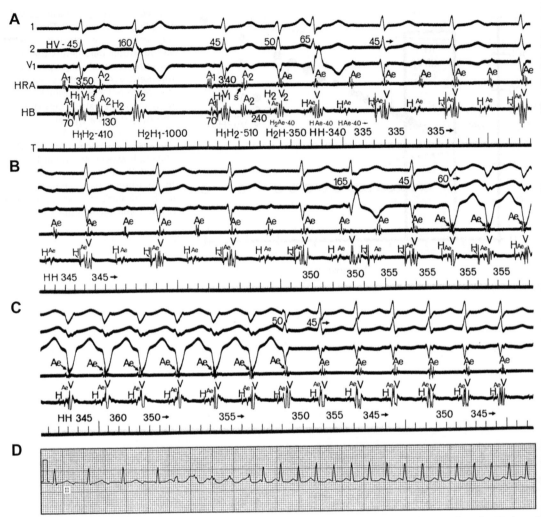

Fig. 61. Atrioventricular (AV) nodal reentry at the His-Purkinje system (HPS). It is well-known that the His bundle and beyond do not participate in AV nodal reentry, so a block in the bundle branches in the HPS will not have any impact on the CL of the tachycardia. However, various HPS occur during these tachycardias and make for interesting electrocardiographs (ECGs). (A) The onset of AV nodal reentry with the second A_2. The first A_2 prolongs AV nodal conduction to 130 and HV interval to 160 the HV intervals are all listed on top of lead II unless they change. The second A_2 shows a marked jump of AH, which is a phenomenon seen with functional duality of AV nodal pathways. This is followed by a brief period of His-Purkinje Wenckebach. Notice the HV of 50, 65, and then block below the His. Subsequent to that there is a 2:1 block below the His. When there is no QRS, one can notice a relatively small duration after the p wave because, as the impulse emerges from the AV node retrograde, it activates both atria at the same time different than sinus beat. In the second panel, the 2 are not continuous. A 2:1 block in the HPS continues and ends with another HPS Wenckebach where the HV is 45, 165, then blocked below the His. Subsequently, 1:1 conduction with a left bundle branch block occurs and continues in the third panel, where it changes to narrow QRS. The phenomena in B and C are also depicted in D on a surface ECG, which starts with a 2:1 block below the His, with 1:1 conduction and a left bundle branch converts to narrow QRS with 1:1 conduction. Throughout this tracing the atrial CL is not affected by all of the phenomena that occur in the HPS.

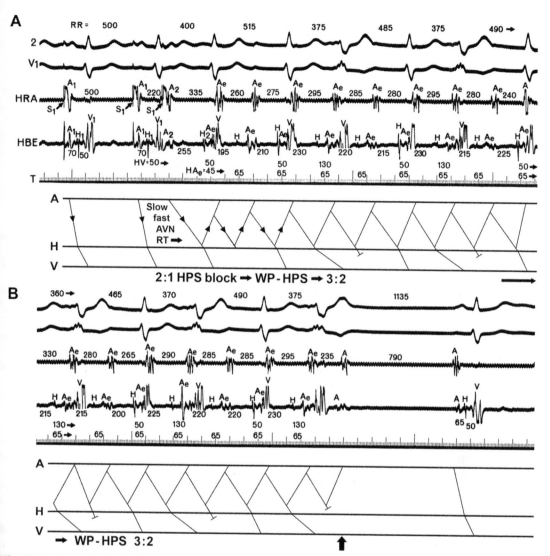

Fig. 62. Atrioventricular (AV) nodal reentry and the His-Purkinje system (HPS). Both *A* and *B* have accompanying letter diagram. The RR intervals are written above lead I. Other pertinent intervals are labeled. The reentry starts with a single premature beat, A_2, and initiates a cycle of 2:1 and 3:2 Wenckebach cycle in the HPS. Note that at the fourth QRS in A, which is narrow, the HV is normal (50 ms). The next HV is 130 and the third H blocks no QRS. This sequence of 3:2 Wenckebach continues. The tachycardia ends with a sudden shortening of AA cycle with the same atrial activation sequence perhaps earlier turnaround in the AV node. The last complex is simply a reference sinus complex. The letter diagrams are self-explanatory.

REFERENCES

1. Rosenbaum MB, Elizari MV, Lazzari JO. Los hemi-bloques. Buenos Aires (Argentina): Paidos; 1968.
2. Fisch C, Zipes DP, McHenry PL. Rate dependent aberrancy. Circulation 1973;48:714–24.
3. Landgendorf R. Atrioventricular and intraventricular block. In: Langendorf R, Pick A, editors. Interpretation of complex arrhyhthmias. Philadelphia: Lea & Febiger (Springer); 1979. p. 217–365.
4. Elizari MV, Lazzari JO, Rosenbaum MB. Phase-3 and Phase 4 intermittent left anterior hemiblock: report of first case in the literature. Chest 1972;62: 673–7.
5. Rosenbaum MB, Lazzari JO, Elizari MV. The role of Phase 3 and Phase 4 block in clinical electrocardiography. In: Wellens HJJ, Lie KI, Janse MJ, editors. The conduction system of the heart: structure, function and clinical implications. Leiden (The Netherlands): HE Stenfert Kroese; 1976. p. 126–42.
6. Rabkin SW, Mathewson FA, Tate RB. Natural history of left bundle branch block. Br Heart J 1980;43:164–9.

7. Flowers NC. Left bundle branch block: a continuously evolving concept. J Am Coll Cardiol 1987;9: 684–97.

8. Auricchio A, Sommariva L, Salo RW, et al. Improvement of cardiac function in patients with severe congestive heart failure and coronary artery disease by dual chamber pacing with shortened AV delay. Pacing Clin Electrophysiol 1993;16:2034–43.

9. Auricchio A, Spinelli J. Cardiac resynchronization for heart failure: present status. Congest Heart Fail 2000;6:325–9.

10. Daubert JC, Ritter P, LeBreton H, et al. Permanent left ventricular pacing with transvenous leads inserted in the coronary veins. Pacing Clin Electrophysiol 1998;21:239–45.

11. Cazeau S, Leclercq C, Lavergne T, et al. Multisite Stimulation in Cardiomyopathies (MUSTIC) Study Investigators. Effects of multisite biventricular pacing in patients with heart failure and intraventricular conduction delay. N Engl J Med 2001;344:873–80.

12. Hardicsay G, Wolkober A. Left bundle-branch block with unfavorable outcomes. Report of Two cases and review of the clinical management and aeromedical decision making. Aeromedical Department CAA, and SALVIMED Medical Services. Budapest (Hungary): National Transport Authority; 2008.

13. Auricchio A, Stellbrink C, Sack S, et al. The Pacing Therapies for Congestive Heart Failure (PATH-CHF) study: rationale, design and endpoints of a prospective randomized, multicenter study. Am J Cardiol 1999;83:130D–5D.

14. Wilkoff BL, Cook JR, Epstein AE, et al, Dual Chamber and VVI Implantable Defibrillator Trial Investigators. Dual-chamber pacing or ventricular backup pacing in patients with an implantable ventricular backup pacing in patients with an implantable defibrillator: the Dual Chamber and VVI Implantable Defibrillator (DAVID) trial. JAMA 2002;288:3115–23.

15. Blanck Z, Georgakopoulos N, Berger M, et al. Electrical therapy in patients with congestive heart failure. Curr Probl Cardiol 2002;27:45–93.

16. Akhtar M, Sra JS. Physiological responses during electrophysiologic evaluation. In: Sra JS, Akhtar M, editors. Practical electrophysiology. Minneapolis (MN): Cardiotext; 2014. p. 39–108.

17. Wellens HJJ, Lie KI, Janse MJ. The conduction system of the heart: structure, function and clinical implications. Leiden (The Netherlands): HE Stenfert Kroese; 1976.

18. Narula OS, Runge M. Accommodation of A-V nodal conduction and fatigue phenomenon in the His-Purkinje system. In: Wellens HJJ, Lie KI, Janse MJ, editors. The conduction system of the heart: structure, function and clinical implications. Leiden (The Netherlands): HE Stenfert Kroese; 1976. p. 529–44.

19. El-Sherif N, Amat-y-Leon F, Schonfield C, et al. Normalization of bundle branch block patterns by distal His bundle pacing. Clinical and experimental evidence of longitudinal dissociation in the pathologic His bundle. Circulation 1978;57:473–83.

20. Narula OS. Longitudinal dissociation in the His bundle. Bundle branch block due to asynchronous conduction within the His bundle in man. Circulation 1977;56:996–1006.

21. Spach MS. Anisotropy of cardiac tissue: a major determinant of conduction? J Cardiovasc Electrophysiol 1999;10:887–90.

22. Wu J, Wu J, Zipes D. Mechanisms of initiation of ventricular tachyarrhythmias. In: Zipes D, Jalife J, editors. Cardiac electrophysiology: from cell to bedside. 4th edition. New York: Saunders (Elsevier); 2004. p. 380–9.

23. Jazayeri M, Deshpande S, Sra J, et al. Retrograde (transseptal) activation of right bundle branch during sinus rhythm. J Cardiovasc Electrophysiol 1993;4:280–7.

24. Sung RK, Kim AM, Tseng ZH, et al. Diagnosis and ablation of multiform fascicular tachycardia. J Cardiovasc Electrophysiol 2013;24:297–304.

25. Kulbertus HE, Demoulin JC. Pathological basis of concept of left hemiblock. In: Wellens HJJ, Lie KI, Janse MJ, editors. The conduction system of the heart: structure, function and clinical implications. Leiden (The Netherlands): HE Stenfert Kroese; 1976. p. 287–315.

26. Dhala A, Gonzalez-Buelgaray J, Deshpande S, et al. Unmasking the trifascicular left intraventricular conduction system by ablation of the right bundle branch. Am J Cardiol 1996;77:706–12.

27. Wenckebach KF. Arrhythmia of the heart: a physiological and clinical study. London: William Green & Sons; 1904.

28. Mobitz W. Uber den partiellen Herzblock. Z Klin Med 1928;107:449.

29. Langendorf R, Cohen H, Gozo EG. Observations on second degree atrioventricular block, including new criteria for the differential diagnosis between Type I and Type II block. Am J Cardiol 1972;29:111–9.

30. Akhtar M. Technique of electrophysiologic evaluation. In: Fuster V, Alexander RW, O'Rourke R, et al, editors. Hurst's the heart. 14th edition. New York: McGraw-Hill, Inc; 2007. p. 932–48.

31. McAnulty JH, Rahimtoola SH, Murphy ES, et al. A prospective study of sudden death in "high-risk" bundle-branch block. N Engl J Med 1978;299:209–15.

32. DiMarco JP, Garan H, Harthorne JW, et al. Intracardiac electrophysiologic techniques in recurrent syncope of unknown case. Ann Intern Med 1981;95 542–8.

33. Jazayeri M, Hempe SL, Sra J, et al. Selective transcatheter ablation of the fast and slow pathways using radiofrequency energy in patients with atrioventricular nodal reentrant tachycardia. Circulation 1992;85:1318–28.

34. Morady F, Higgins J, Peters RW, et al. Electrophysiologic testing in bundle branch block and unexplained syncope. Am J Cardiol 1984;54:587–91.

35. Akhtar M, Shenasa M, Denker S, et al. Role of cardiac electrophysiologic studies in patients with unexplained recurrent syncope. Pacing Clin Electrophysiol 1983;6:192–201.

36. Dessertenne F. La tachycardie ventricularire a deux foyers opposes variables. Arch Mal Coeur Vaiss 1996;59:263–72.

37. Rosen KM, Rahimtoola SH, Gunnar RM. Pseudo A-V block secondary to premature nonpropagated His bundle depolarizations. Documentation by His bundle electrocardiography. Circulation 1970;42:367–73.

38. Pick A, Langendorf R. Recent advances in the differential diagnosis of A-V Junctional arrhythmias. Am Heart J 1968;76:553–75.

39. Scheinman MM, Gonzalez RP, Cooper MW, et al. Clinical and electrophysiologic features and role of catheter ablation techniques in adult patients with automatic atrioventricular junctional tachycardia. Am J Cardiol 1994;74:565–72.

40. Oral H, Strickberger SA. Junctional rhythms and junctional tachycardia. In: Zipes D, Jalife J, editors. Cardiac electrophysiology: from cell to bedside. 4th edition. New York: Saunders (Elsevier); 2004. p. 523–7.

41. Jazayeri M, Akhtar M. Atrioventricular nodal reentrant tachycardia. Cardiol Rev 1993;1(4):200.

42. Josephson M. Supraventricular tachycardia. In: Josephson M, editor. Clinical cardiac electrophysiology: techniques and interpretations. 3rd edition. Philadelphia: Lippincott Williams and Wilkins (Wolters Kluwer); 2002. p. 168–271.

43. Josephson M. Supraventricular tachycardias. In: Josephson M, editor. Clinical cardiac electrophysiology: techniques and interpretations. 4th edition. Philadelphia: Lippincott William & Wilkins (Wolters Kluwer); 2008. p. 175–284.

44. Josephson ME, Kastor JA. Paroxysmal supraventricular tachycardias: is the atrium a necessary link? Circulation 1976;54:430–5.

45. Akhtar M, Jazayeri M, Sra J, et al. Atrioventricular nodal reentry: clinical, electrophysiological and therapeutic considerations. Circulation 1993;88:282–95.

46. Akhtar M, Damato AN, Ruskin JN, et al. Antero-grade and retrograde conduction characteristics in three patterns of paroxysmal atrioventricular junctional reentrant tachycardia. Am Heart J 1978;95:22–42.

47. Nogami A, Naito S, Tada H, et al. Demonstration of diastolic and presystolic Purkinje potentials as critical potentials in a macroreentry circuit of verapamil-sensitive idiopathic left ventricular tachycardia. J Am Coll Cardiol 2000;36:811–23.

48. Maruyama M, Tadera T, Miyamoto S, et al. Demonstration of the reentrant circuit of verapamil-sensitive idiopathic left ventricular tachycardia: direct evidence for macroreentry as the underlying mechanism. J Cardiovasc Electrophysiol 2001;12:968–72.

49. Aiba T, Suyama K, Aihara N, et al. The role of Purkinje and Pre-Purkinje potentials in the reentrant circuit of verapamil sensitive idiopathic LV tachycardia. Pacing Clin Electrophysiol 2001;24:333–44.

50. Nakagawa H, Beckman KJ, McClelland JH, et al. Radiofrequency catheter ablation of idiopathic left ventricular tachycardia guided by a Purkinje potential. Circulation 1993;88:2607–17.

51. Akhtar M, Damato AN, Batsford WP, et al. Demonstration of re-entry within the His-Purkinje system in man. Circulation 1974;50:1150–62.

52. Reddy CP, Slack JD. Recurrent sustained ventricular tachycardia: report of a case with His bundle branches reentry as the mechanism. Eur J Cardiol 1980;11:23–31.

53. Touboul P, Kirkorian G, Atallah G, et al. Bundle branch reentrant tachycardia treated by electrical ablation of the right bundle branch. J Am Coll Cardiol 1986;7:1404–9.

54. Caceres J, Jazayeri M, McKinnie J, et al. Sustained bundle branch reentry as a mechanism of clinical tachycardia. Circulation 1989;79:256–70.

55. Blanck Z, Dhala A, Deshpande S, et al. Bundle branch reentrant tachycardia: cumulative experience in 48 patients. J Cardiovasc Electrophysiol 1993;4:253–62.

56. Narasimhan C, Jazayeri M, Sra J, et al. Ventricular tachycardia in valvular heart disease: Facilitation of sustained bundle branch reentry by valve surgery. Circulation 1997;96:4307–13.

57. Merino JL, Carmona JR, Fernández -Lozano I, et al. Mechanisms of sustained ventricular tachycardia in myotonic dystrophy. Implications for catheter ablation. Circulation 1998;98:541–6.

58. Tchou P, Jazayeri M, Denker S, et al. Transcatheter electrical ablation of right bundle branch. Circulation 1988;78:246–57.

59. Cohen T, Chien W, Lurie K, et al. Radiofrequency catheter ablation for treatment of bundle branch reentrant ventricular tachycardia: results and long-term follow-up. J Am Coll Cardiol 1991;18:1767–73.

60. Blanck Z, Deshpande S, Jazayeri M, et al. Catheter ablation of the left bundle branch for treatment of sustained bundle branch reentrant ventricular tachycardia. J Cardiovasc Electrophysiol 1995;6:40–3.

61. Blanck Z, Sra J, Akhtar M. Incessant interfascicular reentrant ventricular tachycardia as a result of catheter ablation of the right bundle branch: case report and review of the literature. J Cardiovasc Electrophysiol 2009;20:1279–83.

62. Coumel R, Attuel P. Reciprocating tachycardia in overt and latent preexcitation. Influence of functional bundle branch block on the rate of the tachycardia. Eur J Cardiol 1974;1:423–36.

63. Wellens HJJ, Durrer D. Supraventricular tachycardia with left aberrant conduction due to retrograde invasion into the left bundle branch. Circulation 1968;38:474–9.

64. Jazayeri M, Deshpande S, Dhala A, et al. Transcatheter mapping and radiofrequency ablation of cardiac arrhythmias. Curr Probl Cardiol 1994;19:285–396.

65. Tchou P, Lehmann MH, Jazayeri M, et al. Atriofascicular connection or a nodoventricular Mahaim fiber? Electrophysiologic elucidation of the pathway and associated reentrant circuit. Circulation 1988;77:837–48.

66. Klein GJ, Guiraudaon GM, Kerr CR, et al. "Nodoventricular" accessory pathway: evidence for a distinct accessory atrioventricular pathway with atrioventricular node-like properties. J Am Coll Cardiol 1988;11:1035–40.

Part III (Cases)

Rare Cause of Infranodal Block

Anwer A. Dhala, MD, FHRS[a,b,*], Anoop K. Singh, MD, BCh[b]

KEYWORDS

- Timothy syndrome • Long QT syndrome • Infranodal block

KEY POINTS

- The patient exhibits multiple features suggestive of Timothy syndrome, which is a multisystem autosomal-dominant condition with findings that include prolonged QT interval, hand and foot abnormalities, dysmorphic facial features, and mental retardation.
- A 2:1 infranodal atrioventricular block may occassionally be seen in the setting of severely prolonged QT interval.
- Functional nature of atrioventricular block is demonstrated by resumption of 1:1 conduction with changes in heart rate.

CLINICAL HISTORY

B.B.W. was a 36-week gestational-age newborn girl delivered via cesarean section for fetal bradycardia. Fetal echocardiogram had previously identified a small pericardial effusion and biventricular hypertrophy with a small muscular, ventricular septal defect. At 28 weeks, she was noted to have episodes of bradycardia, and fetal magnetography had shown 2:1 atrioventricular (AV) block and a prolonged QT interval. At birth, the baby was noted to be in no acute distress, with an Apgar score of 9 at 1 minute. Heart rate soon after birth was 65 beats per minute. Physical examination revealed micrognathia and fusion of the second, third, and fourth fingers bilaterally as well as fusion of the second and third toes bilaterally. Baseline electrocardiogram (EKG) and subsequent EKG on propranolol is shown.

FINDINGS

Baseline EKG shows sinus rhythm with a sinus rate of 125 bpm (PP interval 480 milliseconds), 2:1 atrioventricular block, and a severely prolonged QT interval of 650 milliseconds (corrected QT interval 678 milliseconds). The PR interval of the conducted beat is normal (110 milliseconds). The nonconducted P wave falls on the beginning of the T wave and about 240 milliseconds before the termination of the T wave. After propranolol and mexiletine are started, the heart rate is 109 bpm (PP interval 560 milliseconds), PR interval is 120 milliseconds, one-to-one AV conduction is present, and QT interval is 480 milliseconds (corrected QT interval 647 milliseconds). However, T-wave alternans is now present (**Figs. 1** and **2**).

DISCUSSION/DIAGNOSIS

The above patient exhibits multiple features suggestive of Timothy syndrome, which is a multisystem autosomal-dominant condition with findings that include prolonged QT interval, hand and foot abnormalities, dysmorphic facial features, and mental retardation. The syndrome is a result of a mutation in L-type calcium channel gene (CACNA1C) leading to a sustained inward calcium current (gain of function) during the plateau phase of the action potential. The degree

[a] Aurora Sinai/Aurora St. Luke's Medical Centers, 2801 W Kinnickinnic River Parkway, Suite 777, Milwaukee, WI 53215, USA; [b] Children's Hospital of Wisconsin-Milwaukee Campus, The Medical College of Wisconsin, 8915 W. Connell Ct, Milwaukee, WI 53226, USA
* Corresponding author.
E-mail address: publishing30@aurora.org

Card Electrophysiol Clin 8 (2016) 743–745
http://dx.doi.org/10.1016/j.ccep.2016.07.005

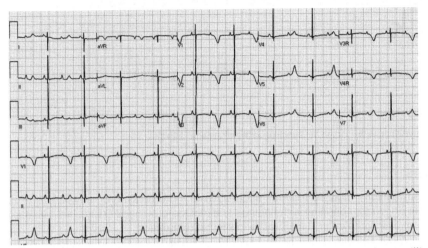

Fig. 1. A 2:1 baseline EKG shows sinus rhythm with a sinus rate of 125 bpm (PP interval 480 milliseconds), 2:1 atrioventricular block, and a severely prolonged QT interval of 650 milliseconds (corrected QT interval 678 milliseconds).

of QT prolongation is usually severe, as it was in this patient.

A 2:1 AV block is seen not only in Timothy syndrome but also in other forms of congenital long QT syndrome as well. Although invasive, electrophysiologic studies were not performed on this patient, and the site of and the functional nature of atrioventricular block can be deduced from the surface EKG. The sinus rate of 125 bpm (cycle length 480 milliseconds) is shorter than the QT interval of 650 milliseconds by 170 milliseconds, and with the addition of the PR interval, the P wave falls well within the QT interval. It can therefore be surmised that the blocked P wave reaches the ventricular muscle during its refractory period. With slowing of the sinus rate, the sinus cycle length is now 560 milliseconds, longer than the QT interval of 480 milliseconds, resulting in the P wave falling outside of T wave, and one-to-one conduction occurs. An alternate explanation for resumption of one-to-one conduction would be shortening of the QT interval sufficiently that the QT interval is

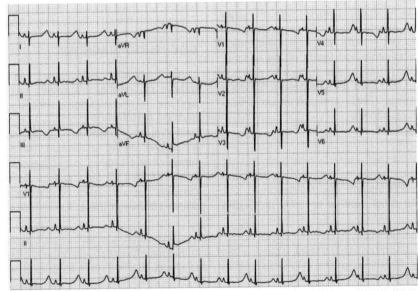

Fig. 2. After propranolol and mexiletine are started, the heart rate is 109 bpm (PP interval 560 milliseconds), PR interval is 120 milliseconds, one-to-one AV conduction is present, and QT interval is 480 milliseconds (corrected QT interval 647 milliseconds).

shorter than the PP interval. At least in this patient, the latter appears unlikely as resumption of 1:1 conduction occurs with significant slowing of the sinus rate and minimal shortening of the QT interval.

Only a few electrophysiologic studies have been carried out in patients with functional 2:1 AV block due to QT prolongation. In probably the first invasive study of such a patient, van Hare and colleagues[1] demonstrated that the block was below the His bundle recording site. Measurements of the ventricular refractory period were obtained by standard electrophysiologic techniques as well as measuring ventricular monophasic action potentials. The functional nature of 2:1 block could be demonstrated by pacing maneuvers that either prolonged or shortened the ventricular refractory period with initiation or resolution of 2:1 block. Other studies have also confirmed that 2:1 block occurs below the His bundle recording site.[2–4] However, there are at least 2 case reports that convincingly demonstrate that infra-Hisian block can also occur in the His-Purkinje network rather than at the level of the ventricular muscle.[2,3] In both of these case reports, the QT interval was only mild to moderately prolonged, and the sinus cycle length was much longer than the QT interval, such that the nonconducted P wave fell outside of the ventricular refractory period, that is, beyond the end of the T wave. Prolonging or shortening the His-Purkinje refractory periods with pacing maneuvers such as short long sequences could induce or terminate 2:1 conduction, confirming the functional nature of infra-Hisian block.

An interesting and potentially significant finding prognostically is also seen when comparing the morphology of the T wave during 2:1 and 1:1 conduction. During 2:1 conduction, the QT interval is constant and the T-wave morphology remains unchanged from beat to beat. With resumption of 1:1 conduction, on the other hand, although the sinus rate is relatively constant, subtle change in the QT interval and obvious T-wave alternans can be appreciated. An excellent explanation for the above findings can be found in a review by Rosenbaum and colleagues.[5] Briefly, the normally seen heterogeneity in action potential duration and restitution kinetics between different layers of the myocardium with abrupt increase in cycle length is greatly exaggerated in patients with prolonged QT. This may have unfortunate consequences, as seen in the case report by Saoudi and colleagues[4] when torsades de pointes degenerating to ventricular fibrillation occurred in a patient with resolution of functional 2:1 block.

The prognosis of 2:1 block associated with long QT syndrome was initially thought to be dire. More recently, the combination of pharmacologic therapy that includes β-blockers, antiarrhythmic drugs to specifically block late sodium current, pacing, and implantable cardioverter-defibrillator therapy have improved the prognosis significantly.

REFERENCES

1. van Hare GF, Franz MR, Rogé C, et al. Persistent functional atrioventricular block in two patients with prolonged QT intervals: elucidation of the mechanism of block. Pacing Clin Electrophysiol 1990;13:608–18.

2. Pruvot E, De Torrente A, De Ferrari GM, et al. Two-to-one AV block associated with the congenital long QT syndrome. J Cardiovasc Electrophysiol 1999;10: 108–13.

3. Lupoglazoff JM, Cheav T, Baroudi G, et al. Homozygous SCN5A mutation in long-QT syndrome with functional two-to-one atrioventricular block. Circ Res 2001;89:E16–21.

4. Saoudi N, Bozio A, Kirkorian G, et al. Prolonged QT, atrioventricular block, and sudden death in the newborn: an electrophysiologic evaluation. Eur Heart J 1991;12:838–41.

5. Rosenbaum MB, Acunzo RS. Pseudo 2:1 atrioventricular block and T wave alternans in the long QT syndromes. J Am Coll Cardiol 1991;18:1363–6.

Review of His-Purkinje System Abnormality with Case Studies

Venkatakrishna N. Tholakanahalli, MD, FHRS[a],*,
Ilknur Can, MD[b], Samuel J. Asirvatham, MD, FHRS[c]

KEYWORDS

- His-Purkinje system • Atrium • Ventricular complex

KEY POINTS

- A single beat arising as extra systole within the His-Purkinje system or from ventricle or even atrium based on conduction timing can invoke delayed conduction or block within intra-Hisian or infra-Hisian sites.
- This may be either manifested in the form of premature atrial or ventricular complexes or concealed as with His extra systoles.
- It appears commonly there is disease within the His-Purkinje system.

INTRODUCTION

Abnormality of the His-Purkinje system (HPS) has varied manifestations ranging from conduction block to extra systoles. HPS abnormality often needs to be invoked to explain paradoxic block at slow heart rates or even the maintenance of block with concealed conduction. The authors present case examples that illustrate the multiple presentation faces of His-Purkinje disease as well as its normal physiology.

Case 1

A 62-year-old male patient presented with symptoms of weakness. His electrocardiogram (ECG) showed 2:1 atrioventricular (AV) block with incomplete right bundle branch block with QRS duration of 120 milliseconds (**Fig. 1**).[1] He was hemodynamically stable with no laboratory abnormalities. The patient underwent electrophysiology study (EPS) to assess the site of conduction block, which showed intra-His and infra-His bundle block

during 2:1 AV block (**Fig. 2**). Further study also demonstrated concealed His-bundle extra systoles (HBE) that caused type I second-degree AV block on the surface ECG, which was due to intra-Hisian Wenkebach conduction (**Fig. 3**).[2]

Calcific or fibrotic lesions in the penetrating region of His bundle, sparing the proximal and distal portions, cause the appearance of split His potentials.[3,4] Patients with intra-Hisian block can present with any type of AV block, but 2:1 AV block is the most frequent presentation.[5] Andrea and colleagues[6] performed EPS of 146 patients presenting with second-degree AV block on surface ECG and found that 16 (11%) of them had intra-His bundle block. Most of their patients with intra-His bundle block were symptomatic and elderly (>60 years) women. In the latter study, all of the patients documented to have intra-His bundle block received permanent pacemaker implantation.

The HBE is considered to be a reflection of diseased HPS. This was apparent in the patient

Disclosures: None for all.
[a] Minneapolis VA Health Care System, University of Minnesota, 111C, One Veterans Drive, Minneapolis, MN 55305, USA; [b] Department of Cardiology, Meram School of Medicine, Necmettin Erbakan University, Konya, Turkey; [c] Mayo Clinic, Rochester, MN, USA
* Corresponding author.
E-mail address: thola001@umn.edu

Card Electrophysiol Clin 8 (2016) 747–752
http://dx.doi.org/10.1016/j.ccep.2016.07.006
1877-9182/16/Published by Elsevier Inc.

cardiacEP.theclinics.com

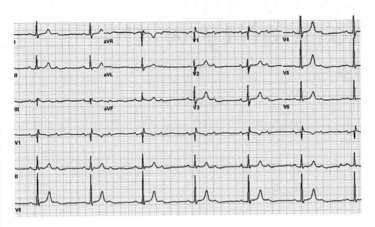

Fig. 1. ECG shows 2:1 AV block. PR interval of the conducted beats is within normal range. (*From* Can I, Guptan A, Li JM, et al. Two-to-one atrioventricular block: what is the mechanism? Heart Rhythm 2009;6: 1526–7; with permission.)

with intra-Hisian block at the baseline in the absence of HBE. The unexpected finding of these depolarizations can manifest as concealed depolarizations, which can lead to sudden appearance of unexplained PR prolongations or type I and type II AV second-degree AV block in the same patient.

Case 2

A 69-year-old man presented to the emergency department with fatigue and dizziness. He was hemodynamically stable, but ECG showed 2:1 AV block (**Fig. 4**A) and Mobitz type I second-degree AV block (see **Fig. 4**B). Laboratory examination including an echocardiogram did not reveal any abnormality. The patient underwent an EPS to determine the site of conduction block. His bundle recordings in **Fig. 4** revealed infra-Hisian Wenkebach and prolonged HV interval. A permanent pacemaker was implanted.

The usual site of type I second-degree AV block (Wenkebach block) is at the level of the AV node. Unless the patient is asymptomatic, pacing is not indicated because progression to advanced AV block is uncommon.[7] Infra-Hisian Wenkebach, on the other hand, is a rare disease reported in only a few cases.[8,9] The patient demonstrated both narrow (see **Fig. 4**) and wide QRS (right bundle branch block; **Fig. 5**) during Wenkebach periodicity, which shows that QRS width is not a reliable indicator of the level of block, AV nodal level versus infra-Hisian. Thus, it is hard to predict the site of AV block in patients with type I second-degree AV block without electrophysiologic testing. The most recent 2012 American College of Cardiology/American Heart Association device-based therapy of cardiac arrhythmias guideline recommends pacemaker implantation for patients with second-degree type I AV block found to be intra-Hisian or infra-Hisian at electrophysiologic study.[10]

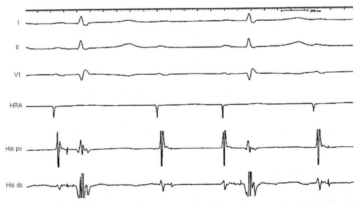

Fig. 2. 2:1 AV block with surface ECG and intracardiac electrograms from high right atrium (HRA), His proxima (His px), and His distal (His ds). His ds electrogram in EPS showed split His potentials in the first A-H-V complex, which is followed by A and single His potential, which is blocked at intra-His and infra-His level. The third beat has intra-His bundle block as well (split His potentials), which is again followed by a blocked sinus beat with intra-His and infra-His level. (*From* Can I, Guptan A, Li JM, et al. Two-to-one atrioventricular block: what is the mechanism? Heart Rhythm 2009;6:1526–7; with permission.)

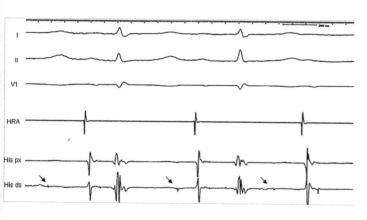

Fig. 3. Type I second-degree AV block on the surface ECG, which was due to concealed His-bundle extra systoles causing intra-Hisian Wenkebach. (*From* Can I, Guptan A, Li JM, et al. Two-to-one atrioventricular block: what is the mechanism? Heart Rhythm 2009;6: 1526–7; with permission.)

Case 3

A 64-year-old male patient with no prior cardiac history presented with his first episode of syncope while he was driving. The patient had normal left ventricular function on echocardiography, and stress test did not show any evidence of ischemia. During his hospitalization, he had episodes of wide QRS complex rhythm captured by telemetry, which was not associated with dizziness or syncope. The patient described them as an abnormal sensation in his chest (**Fig. 6**). An EPS was planned to determine the underlying cause for his syncope. His EPS showed atrial-His interval of 87 and His-ventricular interval of 51 milliseconds. During ventricular stimulation, his wide QRS episodes were easily triggered by premature ventricular stimulations and again terminated by premature ventricular stimulations (**Fig. 7**). The triggered episode when not intervened was nonsustained and was gradually fusing with sinus activation

and terminating (**Fig. 8**). No symptoms were noted during the episode. The wide QRS rhythm appeared to be either right bundle escape versus concealed conduction retrogradely into left bundle with introduction of premature ventricular complex. There was gradual narrowing of QRS indicative of peeling back of refractoriness as the concealment into left bundle moved toward the distal part of the bundle. Adenosine challenge provoked more than 20 seconds of AV block with 24 mg, and despite controversy, may be related to phase IV conduction issue. The findings in the EPS was suggestive of paroxysmal AV block due to phase 4 conduction block in the HPS as potential mechanism for syncope, and a permanent pacemaker was implanted. The patient did not have any further episodes.

Paroxysmal AV block is defined as a sudden pause-dependent phase 4 AV block occurring in the diseased conduction system.[11] Right bundle branch block is the most common baseline distal

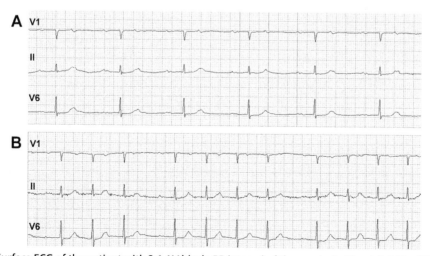

Fig. 4. (*A*) Surface ECG of the patient with 2:1 AV block. PR interval of the conducted beats is 360 milliseconds. (*B*) Same patient demonstrating variable degree of Wenkebach-type second-degree AV block.

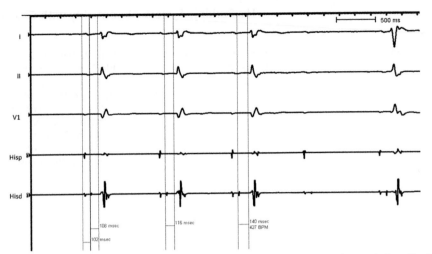

Fig. 5. Surface ECG shows right bundle branch block. Intracardiac electrograms from His bundle showed prolonged HV interval (108 milliseconds). AH interval was 102 milliseconds. The HV interval is prolonged progressively from 108 milliseconds to 140 milliseconds, thereby revealing infra-His Wenkebach and then is followed by infra-His conduction block of the fourth sinus beat.

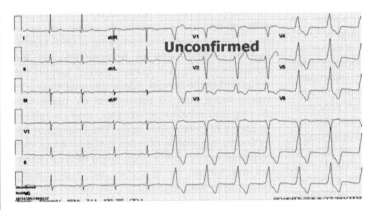

Fig. 6. Spontaneous wide QRS episode initiation after narrow QRS beats.

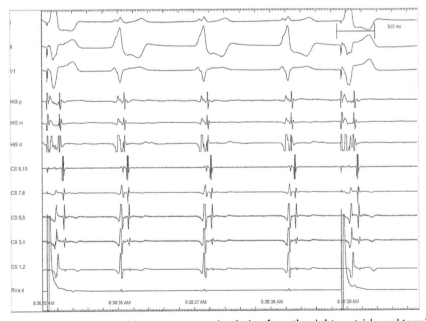

Fig. 7. Wide QRS episode was initiated by a premature stimulation from the right ventricle and terminated again by a premature from the ventricle. CS, coronary sinus; RVa d, right ventricle distal.

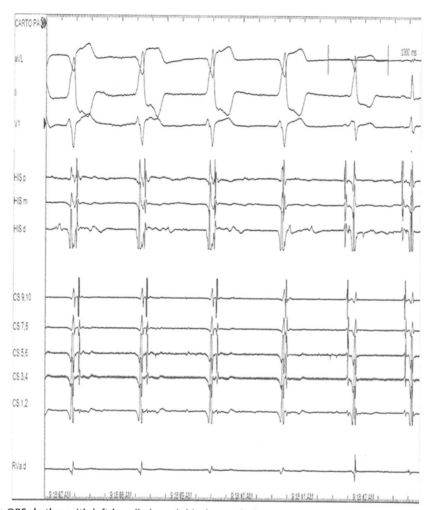

Fig. 8. Wide QRS rhythm with left bundle branch block morphology was initiated with a single premature stimulation from the RV. The episode terminated spontaneously with fusion with sinus activation.

conduction disease. However, Wellens and colleagues[11] reported normal baseline QRS in 28% of the 68 patients of paroxysmal AV block. This patient had a baseline normal QRS as well.

In conclusion, a single beat arising as extra systole within the HPS or from ventricle or even atrium based on conduction timing can invoke delayed conduction or block within intra-Hisian or infra-Hisian sites. This may be either manifested in the form of premature atrial or ventricular complexes or concealed as with His extra systoles. It appears commonly there is disease within the HPS.

REFERENCES

1. Can I, Guptan A, Li JM, et al. Two-to-one atrioventricular block: what is the mechanism? Heart Rhythm 2009;6:1526–7.
2. Narula OS, Scherlag BJ, Samet P. His bundle blocks and his bundle rhythms. Dis Chest 1969;56:238.
3. Rosen KM, Rahimtoola SH, Gunnar RM. Pseudo A-V block secondary to premature nonpropagated His bundle depolarizations: documentation by His bundle electrocardiography. Circulation 1970;42(3):367–73.
4. Bharati S, Lev M, Wu D, et al. Pathophysiologic correlations in two cases of split His bundle potentials. Circulation 1974;49:615–9.
5. Guimond C, Puech P. Intra-His bundle block (102 cases). Eur J Cardiol 1976;4:481–93.
6. Andrea EM, Atie J, Maciel WA, et al. Intra-His bundle block. Clinical, electrocardiographic, and electrophysiologic characteristics. Arq Bras Cardiol 2002; 79:526–37.
7. Strasberg B, Amat-Y-Leon F, Dhingra RC, et al. Natural history of chronic second-degree atrioventricular nodal block. Circulation 1981;63(5):1043–9.
8. Antoniadis AP, Fragakis NK, Maligkos GC, et al. Infra-Hisian block as cause of Wenckebach's phenomenon in an asymptomatic middle-aged man. Europace 2010;12:898–902.

9. Marijon E, Combes N, Boveda S, et al. Wenckebach type block on surface ECG due to infra-Hisian location in a patient with repaired tetralogy of Fallot. Europace 2008;10:641–2.

10. Epstein AE, DiMarco JP, Ellenbogen KA, et al. 2012 ACCF/AHA/HRS focused update incorporated into the ACCF/AHA/HRS 2008 guidelines for device-based therapy of cardiac rhythm abnormalities: a report of the American College of Cardiology Foundation/American Heart Association task force on practice guidelines and the Heart Rhythm Society. J Am Coll Cardiol 2013;61:e6–75.

11. Lee S, Wellens HJ, Josephson ME. Paroxysmal atrioventricular block. Heart Rhythm 2009;6:1229–34.

Bidirectional Ventricular Tachycardia Due to a Mixture of Focal Fascicular Firing and Reentry

Sarfraz A. Durrani, MD[a],*, Raphael Sung, MD[b],
Melvin Scheinman, MD[c]

KEYWORDS

- Bidirectional ventricular tachycardia • Fascicular tachycardia • Bundle branch reentry
- Enhanced automaticity

KEY POINTS

- A 77-year-old man with a history of ischemic cardiomyopathy, hyperlipidemia, and an ejection fraction of 25% presented to the hospital with symptoms of palpitations and shortness of breath and implantable cardioverter-defibrillator shocks.
- In a case of bidirectional ventricular tachycardia (VT) in the setting of ischemic cardiomyopathy and conduction system disease, a unique mechanism of alternating reentry and automaticity was observed, which perpetuated the VT.
- The VT was successfully eliminated with a single lesion at the junction of left anterior fascicle and left anterior superior fascicular.

CLINICAL HISTORY

A 77-year-old man with history of ischemic cardiomyopathy, hyperlipidemia, and an ejection fraction (EF) of 25% presented to the hospital with symptoms of palpitations and shortness of breath and implantable cardioverter-defibrillator (ICD) shocks.[1–24]

He had a past medical history of 2 myocardial infarctions 18 years and 12 years before presentation. He had undergone multiple vessel coronary artery bypass surgery. He underwent an ICD implant several years before presentation for primary prevention. Six years after the ICD implant, in July 2012, he presented to the emergency department (ED) with multiple episodes of ventricular tachycardia (VT), some of which were pace terminated and others required ICD shocks.

He was started on mexiletine, which he discontinued because of nausea and tremors, and was readmitted with multiple ICD shocks with failed anti-tachycardia pacing therapies. On admission he was noted to be in sustained VT, which was just less than his VT detection rate.

The electrocardiogram (ECG) confirmed bidirectional wide complex tachycardia (**Fig. 1**B). Overnight, he remained in stable wide complex tachycardia for several hours. Spontaneous premature ventricular contractions (PVCs) were noted on ECG when he regained sinus rhythm (see **Fig. 1**A).

A second sustained VT was noted at baseline with only right bundle and inferior axis (**Fig. 2**A).

Question: What does the ECG suggest in terms of the mechanism of the wide complex tachycardia?

[a] MedStar Heart and Vascular Institute, #501 Hamaker court, Fairfax, VA 22031, USA; [b] Peninsula Primary Care, Cardiology, 30 Garden Court, Suite B, Monterey, CA 93940, USA; [c] University of California San Francisco Medical Center, 500 Parnassus Avenue, MUE 436, San Francisco, CA 94143-1354, USA
* Corresponding author.
E-mail address: sarfraz.A.Durrani@medstar.net

Card Electrophysiol Clin 8 (2016) 753–764
http://dx.doi.org/10.1016/j.ccep.2016.07.007
1877-9182/16/© 2016 Elsevier Inc. All rights reserved.

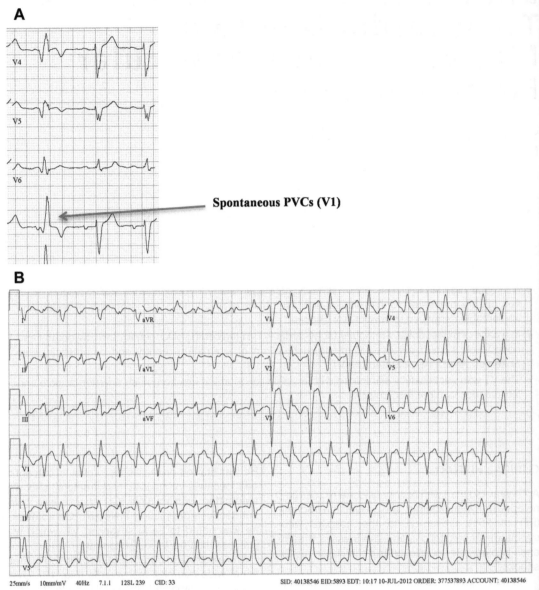

Fig. 1. (*A*) Spontaneous premature ventricular contractions (PVCs) with left posterior fascicle (LPF) block. In sinus rhythm, there were frequent PVCs with the identical morphology to the red bundle branch block (RBBB) pattern seen in tachycardia. The arrow points to PVCs, and a short PR interval confirms the presence of PVCs. (*B*) This image shows a 12-lead ECG with alternating RBBB and LPF block pattern with a left bundle branch block with a right inferior axis.

On *physical examination* he was alert and oriented with rapid heart rates but stable blood pressure (104/58 mm hg). He had a jugular venous distension of +5 cm. There was no murmur, gallop, or rub. Lungs were clear to auscultation; the respiratory rate was 20 per minute; and oxygen saturation was 98% on oxygen. His laboratory test results were normal with a troponin of 0.12, which peaked at 1.4. The chest radiograph did not reveal any acute process.

Two-dimension *echocardiogram* in the hospital showed his EF had now decreased to 15%. A decision was made to proceed with electrophysiology study and ablation of his bidirectional VT (BDVT).

EPS AND RADIO FREQUENCY ABLATION

After informed consents, access was obtained to the right femoral artery and femoral vein. Two

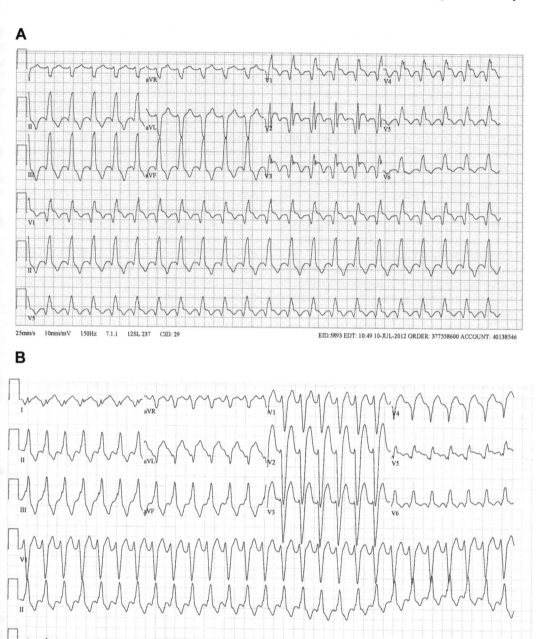

Fig. 2. (A) A 12-lead ECG showing sustained wide complex tachycardia identical to the right bundle branch block pattern seen in **Fig. 1A**. (B) A 12-lead ECG showing wide complex tachycardia identical to left bundle VT pattern in **Fig. 1B**.

quadripolar catheters were advanced and placed in the His and right ventricular (RV) apex locations.

At baseline the patient was in sinus rhythm with a prolonged HV interval and incomplete left bundle branch block.

Spontaneous PVCs identical to the right bundle VT (RBVT) morphology were noted in sinus rhythm (see **Fig. 1A**).

With programmed extrastimuli, VT was easily induced. Three different morphologies of VT were induced: right bundle with inferior axis (see

Fig. 2A), left bundle with inferior axis (see **Fig. 2B**), and a BDVT (see **Fig. 1B**) with alternating left bundle and right bundle morphologies.

At baseline there was evidence of conduction system disease with prolonged HV intervals of 77 milliseconds (**Fig. 3A**).

During VT a clear His potential could not be identified, thus ruling against a right bundle reentry mechanism (see **Fig. 3B**). Overdrive pacing from RV apex was consistent with a different paced morphology than either of the VT morphologies, although postpacing intervals (PPI) were the same as left bundle VT (LBVT). This finding was interpreted as manifest fusion with entrainment of a macroreentrant circuit in close proximity to the ventricular septum (**Fig. 4**).

A propagation map of the VT using 3-dimensional (3D) mapping (CARTO, Biosense Webster), and a 3.5-mm irrigated tip mapping and ablation catheter was created.

Using 3D mapping, the authors constructed activation maps of both the VT circuits separately and then integrated them into one activation map using twice the cycle length of the VT. Both the right and left ventricles were mapped. Before induction of VT, the left anterior fascicle (LAF) was identified in sinus rhythm with a sharp prepotential.

With VT induction, this site (**Fig. 5**) was mapped earliest for right bundle VT (RBVT); the high right septum (anatomic His location) was identified as the earliest activation for the left bundle morphology VT (LBVT), although a prepotential in the left high septum preceded the earliest activation on the right septum (**Figs. 5** and **6**).

Propagation mapping suggested the RBVT propagated from the high left ventricular (LV) septum, the site of previously identified LAF toward the lateral wall of the LV, the LBVT was earliest just distal to this site and broke through across the septum to RV His bundle area.

An early prepotential was identified in the area of LAF. Overdrive pacing was performed at this site, which resulted in capture of LV with a morphology that was identical to the LBVT, moreover the postpacing interval (PPI) was identical to the tachycardia cycle length.

Overdrive pacing from RV apex during LBVT resulted in a different paced morphology but with a good PPI. This suggested the RV apex was close to but not critical to the VT circuit. The authors think this morphology was consistent with a reentrant circuit, which was orthodromic down the left septal fascicle (LSF) and retrograde along the left posterior fascicle (LPF).

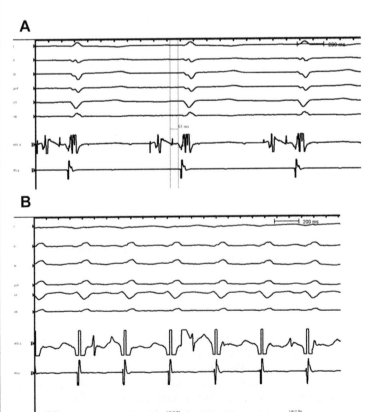

A

B

Fig. 3. (*A*) Prolonged HV (61 milliseconds) at baseline. (*B*) His no longer present during left bundle VT.

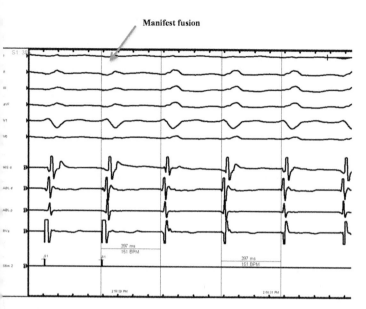

Fig. 4. Overdrive pacing from the mid RV apex consistent with the outer-loop/exit site. BPM, beats per minute.

During BDVT overdrive pacing was performed from LAF (**Fig. 7**), which was identical to the RBVT morphology and the LBVT was also successfully entrained. Pacing was then performed from just septal and distal to the LAF and was thought to capture the LPF (**Fig. 8**). This morphology was now identical to the LBVT with excellent PPI (**Fig. 8**). It was, thus, confirmed that both the circuits were arising at the bifurcation of the LAF and the left anterior superior fascicular (LSF).

Radio frequency (RF) energy was delivered at this site at 30-W output through an irrigated tipped catheter, which resulted in termination of LBVT morphology first and, 30 seconds later, termination of the RBVT morphology as well.

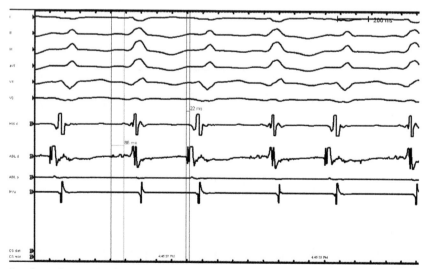

Fig. 5. Recording from the proximal LAF shows a fractionated fascicle potential recorded 86 milliseconds in front of the QRS for the right bundle branch block form and a later potential preceding the QRS 22 milliseconds before the left bundle branch block form. Note that a His bundle recording is absent from either bundle branch pattern, which serves to exclude any supraventricular tachycardia as well as bundle-to-bundle reentry. During LBVT the RV apical recording is much later than the septal ventricular electrogram, which again excludes bundle-to-bundle reentry.

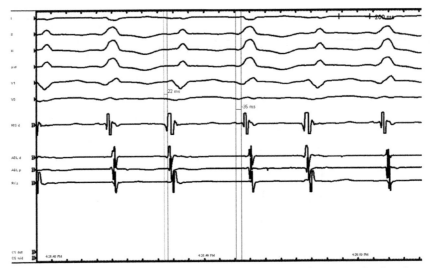

Fig. 6. Mapping the RV during LBBB tachycardia shows that although earliest RV activation site was recorded over the RV septum, this was much later from that recorded from the LV septum during both RB and LB tachycardias (see **Fig. 5**). The much later inscription of the RV apical versus right septal recordings also excludes BBRT because the reverse would be true with the latter.

DISCUSSION

BDVT is a rare phenomenon that is usually attributed to triggered activity as in CPVT or enhanced automaticity as in digitalis toxicity. Rarely, a reentrant mechanism has been invoked to explain BDVT.[20]

Fascicular arrhythmias depend on the specialized conduction system, including the His, right and left bundle, left-sided fascicular bundles, and Purkinje network.

Fascicular tachycardias can arise in structurally normal hearts, with *intrafascicular reentry* being the most common mechanism. These arrhythmias are typically verapamil sensitive. Intrafascicular reentry usually involves the LPF.

Interfascicular reentry and triggered activity or automaticity are additional mechanisms in normal hearts.

The fascicular VT mechanism invoked in the presence of organic heart disease and significant conduction system abnormality is typically

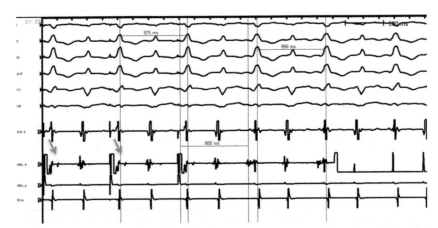

Fig. 7. Overdrive pacing (at twice cycle length) from the region of the LAF shows a right bundle branch block (RBBB) QRS pattern identical to right bundle VT. Also note that the left bundle branch block (LBBB) pattern is accelerated to the paced rate. Hence, overdrive pacing from the LAF reproduces the RBBB pattern and serves to entrain the LBBB pattern to the paced rate. Note the orthodromic entrainment of the fascicle potential, seen only with pacing (*red arrow*). BPM, beats per minute.

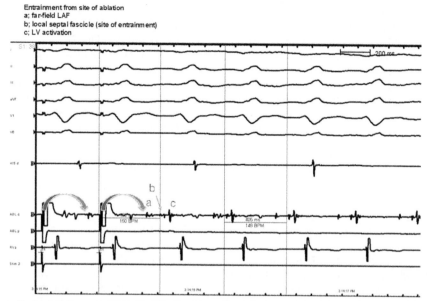

Entrainment from site of ablation
a; far-field LAF
b; local septal fascicle (site of entrainment)
c; LV activation

Fig. 8. Pacing site is slightly septal/distal to **Fig. 7** with earlier LAF potential in LBVT. Ventricular pacing from the LAF fascicle region with prepotential slightly earlier compared with recording site in **Fig. 7**. During sustained left bundle branch block (LBBB) tachycardia, a fascicle potential (b) is recorded well before the QRS. Overdrive pacing from this site shows a paced QRS very similar to the spontaneous tachycardia with orthodromic capture of (b) at the paced cycle length. In addition, note orthodromic capture of potential labeled (a), which is much shorter than the paced cycle length and may be a far field signal or a fascicle potential from a contiguous fascicle, likely LSF. The authors propose that the paced QRS reflects conduction over the septal fascicle and gives an LBBB pattern, which is in close proximity to LAF (see text for discussion).

interfascicular VT, which commonly includes bundle branch reentry and sometimes LAF or LPF. Significant conduction system disease is an important component of interfascicular VT, which allows for stable reentry due to slowed conduction.

This patient had a low EF of 15% at presentation and a prolonged HV interval on EPS; he also had very slow conduction along his LAF.

Recently, interfascicular VT involving the LSF has been described by the authors.[11] In that particular case, VTs of different morphologies were induced during the course of ablation, depending on which limbs of the interconnected specialized conduction system were actively participating during the VT. There are some similarities between the two cases, including that both VT morphologies terminated with RF at the base of LAF.

Anatomic and histopathologic studies of the specialized conduction system have delineated the presence of 3 main fascicles arising from the main left bundle branch (LBB).[23] The LAF and LPF are commonly recognized; in addition, a mid or upper septal fascicle (LSF) has been well characterized anatomically, with a growing body of evidence on the electrocardiographic data

supporting its role in LV conduction.[23–29] Tawara's macroscopic depiction of a trifascicular branch extending out from the LBB in human hearts was the first recognition of the middle or septal fascicle; the LSF anatomy was further established, based on reconstructed histologic transverse sections of the LBB by Demoulin and Kulbertus.[24] Their diagrammatic illustrations of the left-sided conduction system bundles in 20 normal hearts yielded the following findings.

The authors describe as a unique case of BDVT with several important distinguishing features.

This is a BDVT using the specialized conduction system.

The authors think both enhanced automaticity and reentrant mechanisms best explain the arrhythmia.

In this case report, the patient has advanced conduction system disease at baseline, which allows for potential interfascicular reentry. Also, premature ventricular depolarizations are noted in sinus rhythm (see **Fig. 1A**), which have the same morphology as the RBVT. The authors can conclude these to be PVCs rather than aberrantly conducted beats, as the PR interval is very short with these premature beats. They have a right bundle branch block

(RBBB) and right axis deviation (RAD) morphology, consistent with origin in the LAF.

The authors think an automatic tachycardia originates from the proximal LAF, which is in very close proximity to the LSF (**Fig. 9**) and inscribes the sustained RBBB RAD morphology. With conduction down the LAF, typical RB and RAD morphology VT is induced, which can sustain by itself.

Occasionally, the anterograde conduction is blocked in the LAF in a 2:1 fashion and conducts down the septal fascicle in the anterograde direction and LPF in the retrograde direction; the cycle is then repeated and perpetuated.

With programmed extrastimulation, both BDVT and LBVT were induced, confirming the existence of reentrant intrafascicular circuit involving the LPF and LSF.

The RBVT was paced (see **Fig. 7**) from the takeoff of the LAF, which resulted in identical paced morphology and orthodromic conduction of prepotential (LAF). Moreover, the LBVT was accelerated to the paced cycle length. Hence, overdrive pacing

from the LAF reproduces the RBBB pattern and serves to entrain the LBB block (LBBB) pattern to the paced rate (see **Fig. 7**).

For the LBVT the earliest prepotential is seen in the LV near the LAF (see **Figs. 5** and **8**), and the earliest ventricular activation is noted in the basal RV septum about 20 to 30 milliseconds later (white arrow on activation mapping of RV, **Fig. 10**). This site was likely the exit site for the LBVT, but the circuit involves LSF (anterograde) and LPF (retrograde). The authors performed overdrive pacing close to the exit site (upper, mid RV septum); the PPI was short, but the paced morphology was different from VT because of the outer loop exit site proximity (see **Fig. 4**).

The LBVT was also entrained from the putative junction of LAF and LSF, which was just distal to the previous site in the basal LV septum. At this site the prepotentials were earliest and a perfect paced match to LBVT morphology was obtained; the PPI was also the same as the cycle length (see **Figs. 8** and **11**).

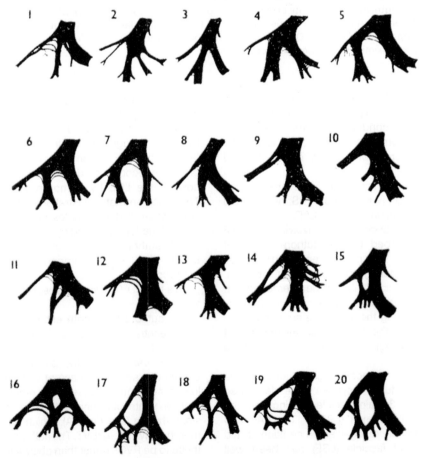

Fig. 9. LV conduction system from 20 normal hearts. (*From* Demoulin JC, Kulbertus HE. Histopathological examination of concept of left hemiblock. Br Heart J 1972;34:807–14; with permission.)

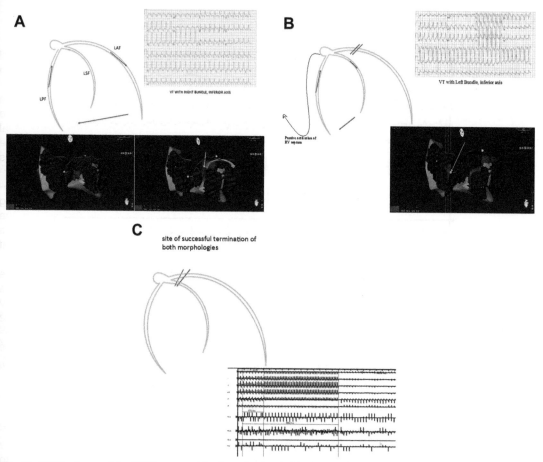

Fig. 10. (*A*) The bases of the RBBB pattern. The impulse (probably due to abnormal automaticity) is conducted antegrade over the LAF and conducted retrograde over the LPF. The activation map shows initial activation of the anterolateral LV. The white arrow shows the site of prepotential and successful ablation. (*B*) The emerging impulse from the LPF is blocked in the LAF and conducts antegrade over the septal fascicle, which emerges in close proximity to the LAF. The septal fascicle activates the central septal area of the LV (note that the earliest activation during LBBB tachycardia was over the basal LV septum [see **Fig. 5**] followed by the RV septum [*white arrow*]). The authors hypothesize that the LBBB pattern was due to early activation of the septum with early RV breakthrough. The bidirectional pattern is due to a 2:1 block in the LAF. (*C*) The authors postulate that the close proximity of LAF and left septal fascicle explain the near simultaneous ablation of both tachycardias with one ablation application.

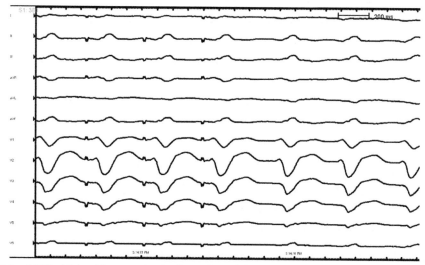

Fig. 11. A 12-lead ECG obtained from pacing in the region of the septal fascicle (LSF), which is nearly identical to the LBVT form.

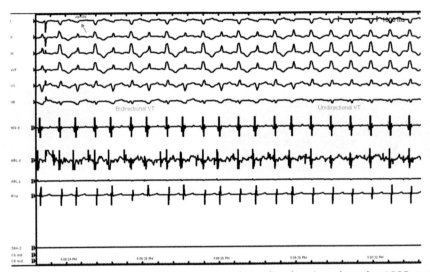

Fig. 12. RF ablation is initiated during bidirectional tachycardia showing that the LBBB tachycardia is ablated first followed by ablation of the RBBB form after 30.5 seconds. The authors interpreted this as the septal and LAF being in close anatomic proximity if not connected to one another. The initial ablation energy seemed to target the septal fascicle, and this subsequently spread to involve the contiguous LAF (see **Fig. 9C**). All arrhythmias were abolished after the initial ablation, and several consolidating ablations were administered.

Concealed entrainment from the LV septum ruled in favor of LSF and LPF circuit with passive RV activation.

At the site of successful ablation and entrainment (see **Fig. 8**) a far field potential (a, LAF) is passively entrained and a local (b, LSF) potential actively entrained.

Ablation at this site results in block in the LSF with termination of LBVT; subsequently, because of the close proximity or in fact connection to one another, the automatic RBVT is also terminated (see **Figs. 10, 12** and **13**).

In more than 3 years of follow-up, the patient has had no recurrence of VT.

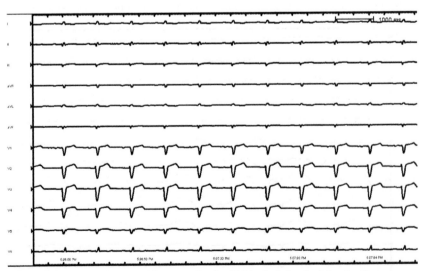

Fig. 13. Sinus rhythm with normal axis and low amplitude QRS in limb leads. Of note, there was no evidence of either RBBB or LBBB.

SUMMARY

In a case of BDVT in the setting of ischemic cardiomyopathy and conduction system disease, a unique mechanism of alternating reentry and automaticity was observed, which perpetuated the VT. The VT was successfully eliminated with a single lesion at the junction of LAF and LSF.

REFERENCES

1. Schwensen C. Ventricular tachycardia as the result of the administration of digitalis. Heart 1922;9: 199–204.

2. Valent S, Kelly P. Digoxin-induced bidirectional ventricular tachycardia. N Engl J Med 1997; 336(8):550.

3. Stubbs WA. Bidirectional ventricular tachycardia in familial hypokalaemic periodic paralysis. Proc R Soc Med 1976;69(3):223–4.

4. Morita H, Zipes DP, Morita ST, et al. Mechanism of U wave and polymorphic ventricular tachycardia in a canine tissue model of Andersen-Tawil syndrome. Cardiovasc Res 2007;75(3):510–8.

5. Berte B, Eyskens B, Meyfroidt G, et al. Bidirectional ventricular tachycardia in fulminant myocarditis. Europace 2008;10(6):767–8.

6. Leenhardt A, Lucet V, Denjoy I, et al. Catecholaminergic polymorphic ventricular tachycardia in children: a 7-year follow-up of 21 patients. Circulation 1995;91(5):1512–9.

7. Levy S, Hilaire J, Clementy J, et al. Bidirectional tachycardia. Mechanism derived from intracardiac recordings and programmed electrical stimulation. Pacing Clin Electrophysiol 1982;5(5):633–8.

8. Levy S, Aliot E. Bidirectional tachycardia: a new look on the mechanism. Pacing Clin Electrophysiol 1989; 12(5):827–34.

9. Rothfeld EL. Bidirectional tachycardia with normal QRS duration. Am Heart J 1976;92(2):231–3.

10. Baher AA, Weiss JN. Bidirectional ventricular tachycardia: ping pong in the His-Purkinje system. Heart Rhythm 2011;8(4):599–605.

11. Sung RK, Scheinman M. Diagnosis and ablation of multiform fascicular tachycardia. J Cardiovasc Electrophysiol 2013;24(3):297–304.

12. Crijns HJ, Wellens HJ. Cure of interfascicular reentrant ventricular tachycardia by ablation of the anterior fascicle of the left bundle branch. J Cardiovasc Electrophysiol 1995;6(6):486–92.

13. Wissner E, Ouyang F. Long-term outcome after catheter ablation for left posterior fascicular ventricular tachycardia without development of left posterior fascicular block. J Cardiovasc Electrophysiol 2012; 23(11):1179–84.

14. Okishige K, Sakurada H, Hirao K, et al. The radio frequency catheter ablation of inter-fascicular reentrant tachycardia: new insights into the electrophysiological and anatomical characteristics. J Interv Card Electrophysiol 2014;41(1):39–54.

15. Nogami A, Iesaka Y. Verapamil-sensitive left anterior fascicular ventricular tachycardia: results of radiofrequency ablation in six patients. J Cardiovasc Electrophysiol 1998;9(12):1269–78.

16. Schmidt B, Ouyang F. Left bundle branch-Purkinje system in patients with bundle branch reentrant tachycardia: lessons from catheter ablation and electroanatomic mapping. Heart Rhythm 2009;6(1): 51–8.

17. Hayashi M, Takano TB. Novel mechanism of postinfarction ventricular tachycardia originating in surviving left posterior Purkinje fibers. Heart Rhythm 2006;3(8):908–18.

18. Okumura Y, Saito S. Idiopathic left ventricular tachycardia with a change from left to right axis deviation during radiofrequency catheter ablation. Int Heart J 2006;47(3):455–60.

19. Lin D, Hsia HH, Gerstenfeld EP, et al. Idiopathic fascicular left ventricular tachycardia: linear ablation lesion strategy for noninducible or nonsustained tachycardia. Heart Rhythm 2005;2(9): 934–9.

20. Ueda-Tatsumoto A, Hiraoka M. Bidirectional ventricular tachycardia caused by a reentrant mechanism with left bundle branch block configuration on electrocardiography. Circ J 2008;72(8): 1373–7.

21. Lopera G, Epstein LM. Identification and ablation of three types of ventricular tachycardia involving the his-Purkinje system in patients with heart disease. J Cardiovasc Electrophysiol 2004;15(1): 52–8.

22. Kuo JY, Tai CT, Chiang CE, et al. Is the fascicle of left bundle branch involved in the reentrant circuit of verapamil-sensitive idiopathic left ventricular tachycardia? Pacing Clin Electrophysiol 2003;26(10): 1986–92.

23. Suma K. Sunao Tawara: a father of modern cardiology. Pacing Clin Electrophysiol 2001;24:88–96.

24. Demoulin JC, Kulbertus HE. Histopathological examination of concept of left hemiblock. Br Heart J 1972;34:807–14.

25. Kulbertus HE. Concept of left hemiblocks revisited. A histopathological and experimental study. Adv Cardiol 1975;14:126–35.

26. Rosenbaum MB, Elizari MV. Left anterior and left posterior hemiblocks. Electrocardiographic manifestations. Postgrad Med 1973;53:61–6.

27. Ibarrola M, Chiale PA, Perez-Riera AR, et al. Phase 4 left septal fascicular block. Heart Rhythm 2014;11: 1655–7.

28. Perrin MJ, Keren A, Green MS. Electrovectorcardiographic diagnosis of left septal fascicular block. Ann Noninvasive Electrocardiol 2012;17:157–8.

29. Perez Riera AR, Ferreira C, Ferreira Filho C, et al. Electrovectorcardiographic diagnosis of left septal fascicular block: anatomic and clinical considerations. Ann Noninvasive Electrocardiol 2011;16:196–207.

Recording the *Accessory His Bundle Potential* from a Right Atriofascicular Accessory Pathway

Warren M. Jackman, MD

KEYWORDS

• His bundle potential • Right atriofascicular accessory pathway • Ventricular preexcitation

KEY POINTS

• *Accessory His bundle potential* (H′) recorded close to the lateral tricuspid annulus during sinus rhythm.
• Increase in A-H′ interval during antidromic atrioventricular (AV) reentrant tachycardia compared with sinus rhythm.
• Early retrograde His bundle (H) potential during antidromic AV reentrant tachycardia (retrograde H recorded <30 milliseconds after QRS onset).

CLINICAL HISTORY

A 42-year-old man with long history of episodes of rapid palpitations.

IMAGING FINDINGS

Fig. 1 shows recordings from the proximal end of a right atriofascicular accessory pathway (RAFP) at the lateral tricuspid annulus (LTA). RAFP represents a duplication of the normal atrioventricular (AV) conduction system with an accessory AV node connected to an accessory His bundle (H′)–right bundle branch (RBBB′), which extends along the endocardial surface of the right ventricular (RV) free wall to fuse with the distal moderator band. In **Fig. 1**A, during sinus rhythm, the LTA$_d$ electrogram shows the local atrial potential (A) followed after 85 milliseconds by an accessory His bundle potential (H′) and the local ventricular potential (V). The normal H and RBB were activated in the antegrade direction.

In **Fig. 1**B, during antidromic AV reentrant tachycardia, the RAFP was activated in the antegrade direction with an additional delay in the accessory AV node (A-H′ increased to 125 milliseconds) due to the increase in rate, as the accessory AV node is responsible for the decremental properties of the RAFP. The RAFP activated the distal moderator band, activating the apical portion of the RV free wall, followed by retrograde conduction over the moderator band and RBB, activating the apical RV septum. The ventricular potential at the tricuspid annulus (LTA$_d$ electrogram) was recorded 25 milliseconds after the onset of the QRS complex, indicating that ventricular activation began far from the base and the atrial end of the atriofascicular pathway. The interval from the H′ to the onset of the QRS was 65 milliseconds and remained fixed despite changes in A-H interval (not shown). Early retrograde activation of the RBB resulted in retrograde RBB (Retro RB) and retrograde H (Retro H) potentials soon after the onset

Heart Rhythm Institute, University of Oklahoma College of Medicine, 1200 Everett Drive, Rm 6E-103, Oklahoma City, OK 73104, USA
E-mail address: warren-jackman@ouhsc.edu

Card Electrophysiol Clin 8 (2016) 765–766
http://dx.doi.org/10.1016/j.ccep.2016.07.008
1877-9182/16/© 2016 Elsevier Inc. All rights reserved.

A   **B**

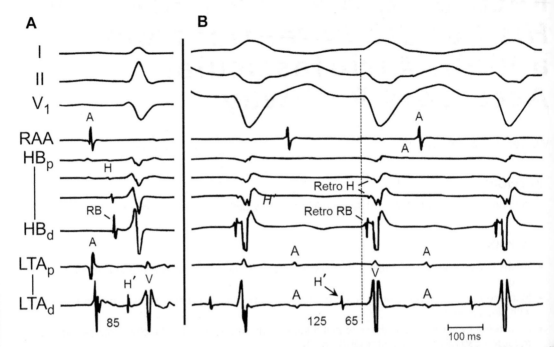

Fig. 1. Recordings from the proximal end of a right atriofascicular accessory pathway (RAFP) at the lateral tricuspid annulus (LTA). (*A*) sinus rhythm. (*B*) antridrome AV re-entrant tachycardia. HB$_p$, proximal bipolar electrogram recorded at His bundle region; HB$_d$, distal bipolar electrogram recorded at His bundle region; LTA$_p$, proximal bipolar electrogram recorded at lateral tricuspid annulus; LTA$_d$, distal bipolar electrogram recorded at lateral tricuspid annulus; RAA, right atrial appendage. (*Modified from* McClelland JH, Wang X, Beckman KJ, et al. Radiofrequency catheter ablation of right atriofascicular [Mahaim] accessory pathways guided by accessory pathway activation potentials. Circulation 1994;89:2655–66.)

of the QRS complex, a characteristic feature of RAFP conduction (retrograde H′ recorded <30 milliseconds after QRS onset). Note the Purkinje like similarity of the H′ in the LTA electrogram to the normal H in the HB electrogram.

PHYSICAL EXAMINATION FINDINGS

The findings were unremarkable.

CLINICAL COURSE

Successful catheter ablation of the right atriofascicular accessory pathway, without recurrence of tachycardia.

Diagnosis/discussion

This information is included in the section on imaging findings.

SUMMARY

This information is included in the section on imaging findings.

FURTHER READING

McClelland JH, Wang X, Beckman KJ, et al. Radiofrequency catheter ablation of right atriofascicular (Mahaim) accessory pathways guided by accessory pathway activation potentials. Circulation 1994;89:2655–66.

Wenckebach Phenomenon in the His-Purkinje System

Masood Akhtar, MD, FACC, FACP, MACP, FAHA, FHRS

KEYWORDS

- Wenckebach phenomenon • His-Purkinje system • Electrocardiogram • Fascicular block

KEY POINTS

- Subtle PR changes may be interpreted as no change, often seen in the His-Purkinje system (HPS) Wenckebach phenomenon (WP).
- Changes in the QRS axis help to localize the site of delay and block along the fibers of fascicles of the left bundle branch.
- Marked PR changes may occur during HPS-WP, which is usually much more subtle. The HV interval changes from 60 milliseconds to 140 milliseconds and then 200 milliseconds before the block.
- All the QRS complexes that are conducted depict right bundle branch and left anterior superior fascicular block, so the visible changes in the HV interval suggest WP mostly occurring in the left posterior inferior fascicle; the complete block of the P wave could be in the His bundle itself or infra-Hissian, that is, the two bundle branches are all 3 fascicles of the left bundle branch.
- Despite obvious HPS-WP, ventricular tachycardia should always be excluded.

PATIENT 1: CLINICAL HISTORY

A 47-year-old woman had experienced palpitations for a year and more recently lightheaded spells. These symptoms were suggestive of a cardiovascular cause. The physical examination was unremarkable. The 12-lead showed sinus rhythm, normal PR interval, and a QRS pattern of right bundle branch block (RBBB) and left anterior superior fascicular (LSF) block.

Workup

Six-lead electrocardiogram (ECG) similar to the previous ECG showed an RBBB and LSF (second and fourth) QRS with further leftward shift during first and third QRS complexes followed by complete block of the P wave. This change occurred without any prior changes in PR or P-P cycle length. These changes suggest Wenckebach phenomenon (WP) in the LSF ending in a complete block of the (second and fifth) P wave. The site of the block in the His-Purkinje system (HPS) was confirmed during electrophysiologic studies (not shown here).

Treatment and Follow-up

Permanent dual-chamber pacing was initiated, and the patient had no further symptoms during the follow-up.

PATIENT 2: CLINICAL HISTORY

This patient is a 78-year-old man with chronic coronary artery disease who was evaluated for recurrent syncope. The left ventricular function

Aurora Cardiovascular Services, Aurora Sinai/Aurora St. Luke's Medical Centers, University of Wisconsin School of Medicine and Public Health, 2801 West Kinnickinnic River Parkway, Suite 777, Milwaukee, WI 53215, USA
E-mail address: Publishing@aurora.org

Card Electrophysiol Clin 8 (2016) 767–768
http://dx.doi.org/10.1016/j.ccep.2016.07.009

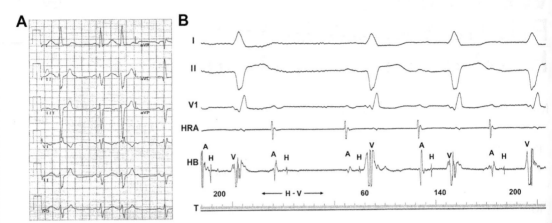

Fig. 1. Two examples of WP in the fascicles of the left bundle branch. Panel (*A*) is in the LSF. Panel (*B*) displays WP in the posterior inferior fascicle. HB, His Bundle; HRA, high right atrial; T, timeline; V, ventricular.

was well preserved (left ventricular ejection fraction 50%). The 12-lead ECG showed sinus rhythm with classic WP (appreciable PR interval lengthening). The QRS showed RBBB morphology and LSF pattern during the conducted complexes raising the possibility of HPS involvement.

Workup

The electrophysiologic evaluation was scheduled for 2 reasons: (1) to confirm the site of block and (2) to rule out ventricular tachycardia (VT). No VT was induced, and the tracing shown depicts that the entire delay and block are localized to the HPS (**Fig. 1**).

Wenckebach Phenomenon in Left Bundle Branch Block

Masood Akhtar, MD, FACC, FACP, MACP, FAHA, FHRS

KEYWORDS

- Wenckebach phenomenon • Left bundle branch block • Electrocardiogram • Tachycardia

KEY POINTS

- The cyclical nature of the event, that is, delay block and normalization, indicates Wenckebach phenomenon (WP) in the left bundle branch block.
- The site of delay and block most likely is in the His bundle suggested by no changes in between His bundle deflection to ventricular deflection (HV), the His deflection and right bundle deflection (HRB), or the right bundle deflection and ventricular deflection (RBV) intervals.
- Loss of Q wave in lead I, even with a narrow QRS, indicates that septal division of the left bundle did not participate in the WP.
- A narrow QRS complex during sinus rhythm and left bundle branch pattern during antidromic tachycardia is the most common clinical presentation in patients with atriofascicular pathways.

CLINICAL HISTORY

A 60-year-old patient had recurrent wide QRS complex tachycardia with a left bundle branch (LBB) and normal axis pattern. The underlying mechanism was atrioventricular nodal reentry tachycardia (AVNRT). Besides the palpitation, there were no other symptoms. The cardiovascular examination was normal.

WORKUP

Most of the workup was directed to the analysis and exclusion of coronary artery disease. The baseline electrocardiogram showed a cyclical pattern with a 3:2 ratio (**Fig. 1**). The two sinus cycles show a LBB block pattern, with a third one being a narrow QRS. During the electrophysiologic (EP) evaluation it was noted that the same 3:2 pattern persisted. The HV interval was prolonged at 70 milliseconds with RBV of 25 milliseconds. Therefore, the His-Purkinje System (HPS) delay seems proximal at least on the right side (HRB = 45 milliseconds). Previously documented supraventricular tachycardia was repeatedly induced, and no other abnormalities were detected. The distinction is made during description of key points between left bundle branch block (aberrant conduction) versus antidromic tachycardia related to atriofascicular pathway by the absence of H(His) deflection before the QRS in the latter case.

Aurora Cardiovascular Services, Aurora Sinai/Aurora St. Luke's Medical Centers, University of Wisconsin School of Medicine and Public Health, 2801 West Kinnickinnic River Parkway, Suite 777, Milwaukee, WI 53215, USA
E-mail address: Publishing@aurora.org

Card Electrophysiol Clin 8 (2016) 769–770
http://dx.doi.org/10.1016/j.ccep.2016.07.010
1877-9182/16/© 2016 Elsevier Inc. All rights reserved.

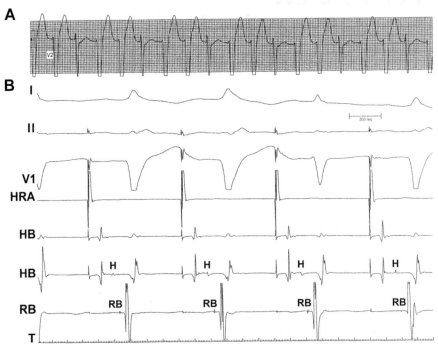

Fig. 1. Wenckebach phenomenon in left bundle branch block. The pattern of 3:2 of Wenckebach phenomenon in the left bundle is shown on rhythm strip (*A*) as well as intracardiac tracing recording (*B*). HB, His bundle; HRA, high right atrial; RB, right bundle; T, timeline.

TREATMENT

Ablation of the supraventricular tachycardia, that is, the slow pathway, was accomplished with elimination of AVNRT and relief of symptoms. Wenckebach phenomenon in the LBB was not associated with any symptoms and did not require any treatment.

FURTHER READING

Narula OS. Longitudinal dissociation in the His bundle. Bundle branch block due to asynchronous conduction within the His bundle in man. Circulation 1977; 56:996–1006.

Retrograde Concealed Conduction in the His-Purkinje System

Masood Akhtar, MD, FACC, FACP, MACP, FAHA, FHRS

KEYWORDS

- His-Purkinje System • Syncope • Premature ventricular complex

KEY POINTS

- Only limited information is available on occasion but can still be useful.
- The block site of a complex can often be detected by its effect on the subsequent complex, as seen in this tracing.
- A long HV that is more than 100 ms in patients with recurrent unexplained syncope and no other obvious cause should receive permanent pacemakers.

CLINICAL HISTORY

An 83-year-old male patient with no cardiovascular pathology was seen due to recurrent syncopal episodes. The 12-lead electrocardiogram showed sinus rhythm, a long PR, and right bundle branch block pattern. The QRS axis was normal.

WORKUP

A complete electrophysiologic examination was planned but was not possible because of access problems. Therefore, only the His bundle recording was obtained with difficulty and the tracing shown here was the best possible His bundle recording (**Fig. 1**).

The analysis of the recording shows sinus rhythm and long PR. Both components of the PR, that is, AH and HV, are prolonged. A spontaneous, premature ventricular beat occurs, which clarifies and validates the His-Purkinje System (HPS) as the site of conduction delay. It can be noted that the premature ventricular complex, which is not followed by either the His deflection or any other signal, has an impact on the subsequent sinus complex. Although the AH remains unchanged, the HV further prolongs, indicating, thereby, that the ventricular premature complex blocked retrogradely in the HPS (concealed conduction). This provides further proof of markedly diseased HPS in a patient with recurrent syncope.

TREATMENT

A permanent dual-chamber pacemaker was implanted with no further syncopal episodes.

Aurora Cardiovascular Services, Aurora Sinai/Aurora St. Luke's Medical Centers, University of Wisconsin School of Medicine and Public Health, 2801 West Kinnickinnic River Parkway Suite 777, Milwaukee, WI 53215, USA
E-mail address: Publishing@aurora.org

Card Electrophysiol Clin 8 (2016) 771–772
http://dx.doi.org/10.1016/j.ccep.2016.07.011
1877-9182/16/© 2016 Elsevier Inc. All rights reserved.

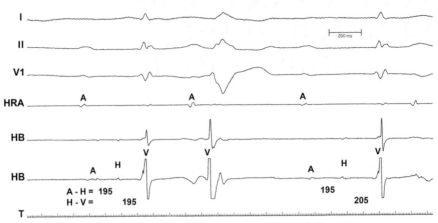

Fig. 1. Concealed conduction in the HPS. A, atrial; H, His bundle; V, ventricular electrograms.

Changes in the Reentrant Pathway in Verapamil-Sensitive Fascicular Reentrant Ventricular Tachycardia During Ablation

CrossMark

Patrick Tchou, MD*, Khaldoun Tarakji, MD, MPH, Mohamed Kanj, MD

KEYWORDS

- Verapamil • Reentrant ventricular tachycardia • Ablation • Case study
- Fascicular activation patterns

KEY POINTS

- This case demonstrates that fascicular reentrant tachycardias can generate different QRS morphologies depending on the path of breakout into the myocardium.
- Ablation of 1 exit path may results in propagation over other fascicular paths.
- Changes in fascicular activation patterns causing changes in cycle lengths demonstrates the reentrant nature of this tachycardia.

CLINICAL HISTORY

A 58-year-old woman with a previously noted structurally normal heart presents to the emergency department with a sustained tachycardia. **Fig. 1** shows the 12-lead electrocardiogram (ECG) of the tachycardia. Intravenous adenosine, lidocaine, and amiodarone infused in the emergency department failed to affect the tachycardia. Cardioversion of the tachycardia resulted in sinus rhythm for a few beats followed by recurrence of the tachycardia. The patient was then admitted to the intensive care unit. The ECG findings were noted to be typical of a verapamil-sensitive ventricular tachycardia (VT). Transient termination of the tachycardia could be achieved with boluses of verapamil. However, even at maximally tolerated infusions of verapamil, the tachycardia would not terminate. The patient was thus taken to the electrophysiology laboratory for mapping and ablation.

ELECTROPHYSIOLOGY STUDIES AND ABLATIONS

The tachycardia was incessant and can only be slowed with large doses of verapamil, which also caused it to become irregular in rate. Mapping of the tachycardia identified early activation near the inferior septal portion of the left ventricle where a fascicular potential preceded ventricular activation (**Fig. 2**). Ablation at this site terminated the tachycardia. A 12-lead of sinus rhythm after ablation is shown in **Fig. 3**.

In sinus rhythm, ventricular function was noted to be markedly depressed. This was attributed to the prolonged and incessant nature of the presenting tachycardia. Verapamil was discontinued and the patient was observed clinically. Within 24 hours, the patient had recurrence of a similar tachycardia. However, now the tachycardia had an inferior axis. The patient was then again taken urgently to the electrophysiology laboratory for

Department of Cardiovascular Medicine, Cleveland Clinic Main Campus, Mail Code J2-2, 9500 Euclid Avenue, Cleveland, OH 44195, USA
* Corresponding author.
E-mail address: TCHOUP@ccf.org

Card Electrophysiol Clin 8 (2016) 773–777
http://dx.doi.org/10.1016/j.ccep.2016.08.001
1877-9182/16/© 2016 Elsevier Inc. All rights reserved.

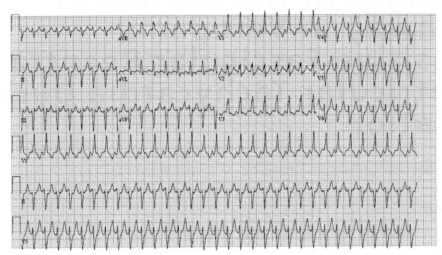

Fig. 1. The presenting 12-lead electrocardiogram with a 3-lead rhythm strip. This shows a tachycardia having a cycle length of 310 ms. The QRS has a right bundle branch block morphology with a superior axis typical of a verapamil sensitive ventricular tachycardia. Ventriculoatrial dissociation is noted in lead V1.

another mapping and ablation procedure. A 12-lead ECG comparison of the baseline tachycardia with the recurrent one is shown in **Fig. 4**. Although the QRS of the recurrent VT maintained a right bundle branch block pattern in V1, its duration was distinctly shorter and its axis had shifted inferiorly.

Mapping in the left ventricle now showed early activation in the anterior wall and an early fascicular potential was identified in the anterior septal region, which activated 45 ms before earliest ventricular activation. The effects of ablation at this site is shown in **Fig. 5**. During application of radiofrequency energy, there was a transition of the QRS

morphology over 3 beats from the right bundle branch block QRS to a left bundle branch block pattern having a much longer QRS duration. The cycle length of the tachycardia slowed by 20 ms with this transition and there was prolongation of the fascicular potential to local ventricular activation interval noted on the ablation tip electrode.

Further mapping more inferiorly along the proximal septum identified earlier fascicular potentials and ablation at this site terminated the tachycardia. No further recurrence of the tachycardia occurred. Her 12-lead ECG then showed a conduction defect with a QRS duration of 114 ms, **Fig. 6**. The HV interval was 50 ms in sinus rhythm.

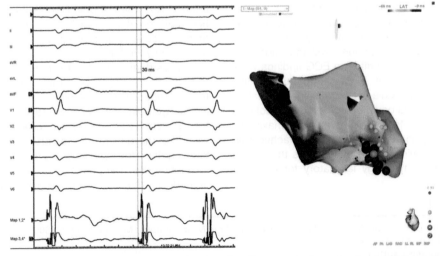

Fig. 2. (*Left*) Intracardiac electrocardiograms at the site of earliest ventricular activation in tachycardia where radiofrequency energy delivery terminated the tachycardia. (*Right*) Right lateral view of CARTO map indicating site of ablation lesions delivery.

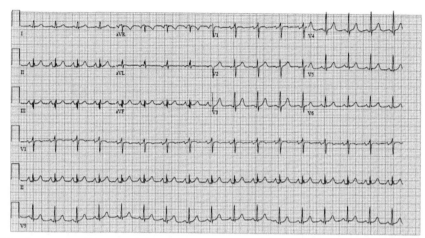

Fig. 3. A 12-lead electrocardiogram of sinus rhythm after successful termination of tachycardia during first ablation.

The patient's ventricular function normalized when assessed by echocardiography 2 months later.

DISCUSSION

This case demonstrates the reentrant nature of this type of tachycardia. **Fig. 7** shows the sequence of events that likely occurred during the application of the various radiofrequency lesions. The reentrant site of the tachycardia likely involved a slowly conducting, verapamil-sensitive tissue connecting to the fibers along the inferior septal portion of the inferior fascicle (see **Fig. 7** left panel). The initial ablation lesions were likely

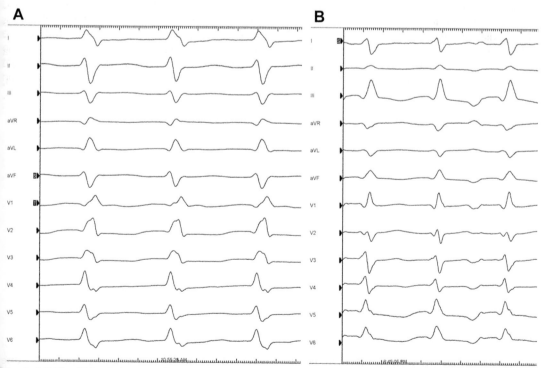

Fig. 4. (*A*) The 12-lead electrocardiogram (ECG) of the tachycardia as recorded during the baseline electrophysiology study before the first ablation. (*B*) The 12-lead ECG of the recurrent tachycardia. Note the change of axis from a superior one at baseline to an inferior one in the recurrent one. Note also the shorter QRS duration in the recurrent ventricular tachycardia.

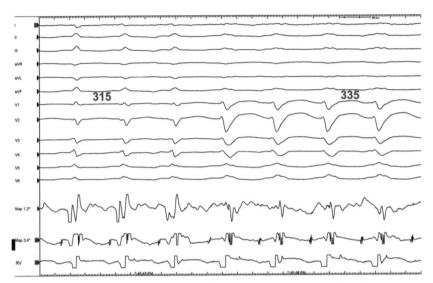

Fig. 5. Effects of ablation at the anterior septal site on the recurrent tachycardia. Note the change in cycle length of the tachycardia associated with transition to a left bundle branch block QRS morphology and the prolongation of the Purkinje potential to local ventricular activation (Map 1,2*) time (+60 ms) and negligible increase in Purkinje potential to RV activation interval (<10 ms).

applied close enough, but distal to the reentry site that they stunned the reentry site and terminated the tachycardia. Although the tachycardia was incessant and recurred immediately post cardioversion even on the maximum tolerated infusion of verapamil, the first ablation terminated the tachycardia and the patient remained in sinus rhythm for near 24 hours. However, either owing to waning of the verapamil effect in some of these slowly conducting tissues or owing to recovery of

conduction in the same tissues, the tachycardia was able to resume. The initial lesions were likely delivered slightly distal to the site of connection into the inferior fascicle. Thus, the distal conduction pathway from the connecting site remained blocked. However, with recovery, the reentrant impulse was able to now conduct retrogradely up the inferior fascicle and then down the anterior fascicle as well as up to the His bundle and down the right bundle. This pattern of ventricular activation

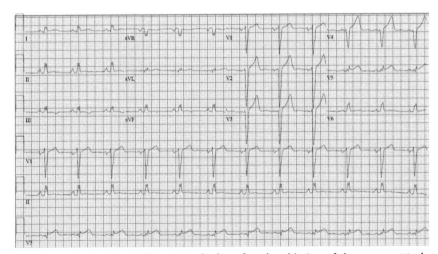

Fig. 6. A 12-lead electrocardiogram (ECG) in sinus rhythm after the ablation of the recurrent tachycardia. Note the intraventricular conduction defect that is new in comparison with the ECG after the first ablation, where the QRS was more narrow. The axis is inferior. These changes in the ECG suggest that there was ablation of a portion of the left sided fascicles, but likely preservation of either the septal of some of the anterior divisions of the left bundle.

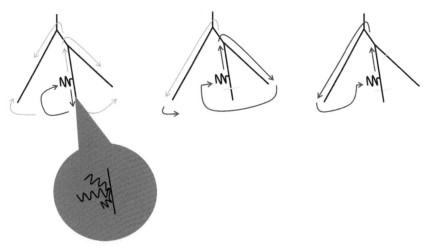

Fig. 7. Sequence of reentrant circuits after application of radiofrequency lesions at different sites along the His–Purkinje system. See discussion in text for details.

resulted in a right bundle branch block pattern as the left ventricle was activated earlier via the left anterior fascicles. But, the QRS was narrower than the baseline VT, because the right bundle was now able to contribute more to right ventricular activation, even though that activation was somewhat delayed in comparison with the activation via the left anterior fascicle. This ventricular activation is illustrated in **Fig. 7**, middle panel. During the second ablation, the initial set of lesions were delivered near the anterior fascicle as the operators suspected a separate anterior fascicular reentrant tachycardia based on the QRS morphology of the VT (right bundle branch block and inferior axis). However, with ablation of the anterior fascicle, the reentrant circuit now only propagated retrogradely up to the His bundle and down the right bundle creating a left bundle branch block QRS for the tachycardia (see **Fig. 7**, right panel). At the same time, owing to the longer pathway for the reentry, the tachycardia slowed by 20 ms. This prolongation is quite consistent with transeptal propagation time. This sequence of events is not compatible with a focal mechanism of tachycardia. Although changes in QRS morphology owing to different pathways of breakout are feasible with a focal mechanism, a change in cycle length owing to block along one of those pathways is unlikely to occur with such a mechanism. Neither are these sequences of changes in the tachycardia consistent with a microreentrant mechanism involving a septal reentry within the fascicles. The fact that creation of an LBBB pattern during the tachycardia slowed the tachycardia cycle length by 20 ms would implicate the local myocardium around the slowly conducting tissue as part of the reentrant circuit. The activation of that myocardium would be delayed

when the LBBB pattern developed. Thus, the sequence of observed changes in this case with the series of applied radiofrequency lesions indicates that the slowly conducting, verapamil-sensitive tissue formed the reentrant circuit and connected from the myocardium to the inferior fascicle near the inferior septal site of the first ablation lesions. The final set of lesions could have ablated the actual insertion site of the slowly conducting tissue. However, the site of these final lesions was higher up along the septum and not at all close to the site of the first set of ablation lesions. Thus, it is more likely that the final set of ablation lesions eliminated the retrograde posterior fascicular path through which the reentrant circuit propagated up to the His bundle.

Although this case was instructive in the nature of the reentrant circuit in this patient, the ablation approach was clearly not optimal. Had the first set of lesions eliminated the connection of the slowly conducting tissue into the fascicle without recovery, these repeated ablations would not have been necessary. However, the repeated ablations applications provided valuable insight into the nature of the reentrant circuit involve in the tachycardia.

SUMMARY

The sequence of changes in the QRS morphology and the accompanying cycle lengths of the tachycardia confirm that the reentrant circuit involves the left ventricular myocardium as well as the His Purkinje system as part of the reentrant circuit. The reentrant propagation likely goes from local left ventricular myocardium into a slowly conducting, verapamil sensitive tissue which then connects into the inferior fascicle.